Cardiovascular Emergencies in Adults

Immediate Management and Advanced Interventions

Dr. Jack F. McDevitt,MD

Acknowledgments

I wish to express my sincere gratitude to my esteemed colleagues, mentors, and the broader community of healthcare professionals whose expertise and commitment to advancing emergency cardiovascular care have profoundly influenced this work. Your invaluable contributions and dedication to excellence have been a constant source of inspiration.

I am especially grateful to my family and friends for their unwavering encouragement and support throughout the development of this manuscript. Their belief in this endeavor has been instrumental in bringing this project to fruition.

Dr. Jack F. McDevitt, MD

Preface

Cardiovascular emergencies are among the most time-sensitive and critical challenges faced by healthcare professionals. The ability to recognize, diagnose, and intervene effectively during these situations can significantly impact patient outcomes, often being the difference between life and death. Cardiovascular Emergencies in Adults: Immediate Management and Advanced Interventions is designed to provide a comprehensive yet practical guide for clinicians navigating the complex landscape of acute cardiovascular care.

The goal of this book is to bridge the gap between theory and practice by offering evidence-based strategies and step-by-step approaches to managing cardiovascular emergencies in adults. It caters to a broad audience, including emergency medicine physicians, cardiologists, internists, advanced practice providers, nurses, and trainees who encounter such cases in their professional practice.

This text delves into the pathophysiology, clinical presentations, diagnostic approaches, and treatment modalities for a wide range of cardiovascular emergencies. From acute coronary syndromes and arrhythmias to cardiogenic shock and hypertensive crises, each chapter provides detailed insights supported by the latest clinical guidelines and research. Practical algorithms and case-based scenarios further enhance the reader's ability to make informed decisions under pressure.

Special emphasis is placed on advanced interventions, including the use of cutting-edge technologies such as extracorporeal membrane oxygenation (ECMO), percutaneous coronary interventions (PCI), and mechanical circulatory support devices. Recognizing the importance of interdisciplinary collaboration, this book also explores the integration of care across emergency departments, intensive care units, and cardiac catheterization labs.

This work is the culmination of years of clinical experience, research, and collaboration with experts across various specialties. It reflects a commitment to empowering healthcare professionals with the knowledge and tools they need to deliver optimal care in critical situations.

As you embark on this journey through the complexities of cardiovascular emergencies, I hope this book will serve as a valuable resource in enhancing your clinical expertise and improving patient outcomes.

Dr. Jack F. McDevitt, MD

Acknowledgement
Preface
Table of content
List of Abbreviations

Table of contents

Chapter 1: Chest Pain

1. Introduction
   - Overview of Chest Pain as a Prototypical Emergency Issue
   - Importance of Risk Stratification and Clinical Judgment

2. Epidemiology
   - Prevalence of Chest Pain in Emergency Departments
   - Trends in Acute Chest Pain Incidences
   - Shifting Patterns in Acute Coronary Syndrome (ACS) Presentations

3. Differential Diagnosis and Approach
    - Life-Threatening Causes
    - Non-Cardiac Causes:
    - Role of Risk Factors in Clinical Assessment

4. Clinical Features
    - High-Risk Indicators for Serious Pathology
    - Common Presentations of ACS, PE, and Aortic Dissection
    - Signs of Non-Cardiac and Musculoskeletal Chest Pain

5. Clinical Investigations
    - Role of ECG in Diagnosing Chest Pain Causes
    - High-Sensitivity Troponin (hsT) Testing and Interpretation
    - Chest Radiographs and Advanced Imaging in Diagnosis

6. Risk Stratification Tools
    - TIMI, HEART, and EDACS Scores

- Evidence-Based Protocols for ACS Management
- Special Considerations for High-Risk Populations

7. Management and Treatment
   - Early Interventions for ACS
   - Tailored Treatment for Non-Cardiac Causes
   - Addressing Non-Specific Chest Pain and Risk Factors

8. Disposition and Prognosis
   - Admission Criteria for High-Risk Patients
   - Discharge Planning and Follow-Up Recommendations
   - Long-Term Outcomes Based on Underlying Conditions

Chapter 2: Acute Coronary Syndromes

1. Introduction to Acute Coronary Syndromes (ACS)
   - Definition and types of ACS

- Advances in diagnostic criteria.

2. Risk Assessment in ACS
   - Formal protocols
   - Accelerated diagnostic protocols (ADAPT).
   - Cardiovascular risk factors and emerging insights.

3. Pathophysiology of ACS
   - Mechanisms of atheroma rupture and thrombus formation.
   - Role of non-atherosclerotic causes
   - Impact of occlusion location on clinical outcomes.

4. Epidemiology
   - Trends in CHD mortality.
   - Age and gender variations in acute coronary event rates

5. Clinical Features
   - Symptomatology of ACS versus other causes of chest pain.

- Differentiating stable angina from ACS.
- Importance of physical examination in complications.

6. Diagnosis of ACS
   - Role of the 12-lead ECG in diagnosis.
   - Use of Sgarbossa criteria in LBBB cases.
   - Biomarkers and other diagnostic tools.

7. Management of STEMI
   - Reperfusion strategies: PCI vs. thrombolysis.
   - Timing of intervention.

8. Management of NSTEACS
   - Clinical pathways and interdisciplinary collaboration.
   - Risk-benefit assessment for antithrombotic therapies.

9. Pharmacological Interventions
   - Antiplatelet agents
   - Antithrombin therapies

- Role of β-blockers, glycoprotein IIb/IIIa inhibitors, and direct thrombin inhibitors.

10. Patient Disposition
    - Admission protocols
    - Criteria for cardiac catheterization or CABG.

11. Common Complications in ACS
    - Arrhythmias and conduction disturbances.
    - Pericarditis.
    - Acute left ventricular failure and cardiogenic shock.
    - Thromboembolism and mechanical complications.

Chapter 3: Acute Pulmonary Oedema (APO)

1. Introduction
    - Overview and significance
    - Definition and clinical presentation
    - Pathophysiology

2. Aetiology and Pathophysiology
    - Cardiogenic APO
    - Non-cardiogenic APO
    - Fluid maldistribution vs. fluid overload

3. Clinical Assessment
    - Patient history
    - Physical examination findings
    - Key diagnostic features

4. Clinical Investigations
    - Electrocardiogram (ECG)
    - Imaging
    - Blood Tests
    - Oximetry

5. Treatment Approaches
    - General Principles
    - Non-Cardiogenic APO
    - Cardiogenic APO:
    - Management in normotensive or hypertensive patients
    - Ventilatory support
    - Pharmacotherapy

6. Management of Hypotension in APO
    - Identification of cardiogenic shock
    - Ventilatory and hemodynamic support
    - Inotropic and vasopressor therapy
    - Advanced interventions

7. Role of Non-Invasive Ventilation (NIV)
    - CPAP vs. BiPAP: Indications and effectiveness
    - Emerging modalities like high-flow nasal cannula (HFNC)

8. Controversies and Emerging Trends
    - Diagnostic challenges
    - Debate on diuretic dosing and vasodilator efficacy
    - New pharmacological agents and their limitations

9. Conclusion
    - Summary of effective management strategies
    - Future directions in APO management

Chapter 4: Arrhythmias

1. Introduction
    - Definition and Classification of Arrhythmias
    - Hemodynamic Stability and Clinical Priorities
    - Management Objectives

2. Pathophysiology and Pathogenesis
    - Normal Cardiac Conduction System
    - Mechanisms of Arrhythmias
    - Abnormal Impulse Generation
    - Abnormal Impulse Conduction
    - Ectopic Impulses
    - Re-entry Mechanisms
    - Enhanced and Abnormal Automaticity
    - Triggered Activity

3. Principles of Assessment and Management
    - Symptom Recognition and Stabilization
    - Investigations: ECG, Blood Tests, Imaging

- Management Strategies

4. Bradyarrhythmias
   - Sinus Bradycardia
   - Causes, Clinical Features, and Management
   - Sick Sinus Syndrome
   - ECG Findings and Treatment
   - Heart Block
   - First-Degree AV Block
   - Second-Degree AV Block (Mobitz Type I and II)
   - Third-Degree (Complete) AV Block

5. Tachyarrhythmias
   - Diagnostic Approach to Tachyarrhythmias
   - Ventricular Tachycardias (VT)
   - Monomorphic VT: Diagnosis and Management
   - Polymorphic VT: Including Torsades de Pointes
   - Supraventricular Tachycardias (SVT)

6. Advanced Management Techniques

- Cardioversion and Pacing
- Pharmacological Interventions
- Long-Term Monitoring and Prevention

7. Figures and Illustrations
    - Conduction System of the Heart
    - ECG Patterns of Arrhythmias
    - Heart Block and Tachyarrhythmia Examples

8. Multifocal Atrial Tachycardia (MAT)
    - Definition and Clinical Features
    - ECG Characteristics
    - Associated Conditions
    - Management Strategies

9. Trifascicular Blocks
    - Overview and Classification
    - ECG Patterns
    - Left Anterior Fascicular Block (LAFB)
    - Left Posterior Fascicular Block (LPFB)
    - Right Bundle Branch Block (RBBB)
    - Clinical Implications and Management

10. Left Bundle Branch Block (LBBB)
- Pathological Associations
- Key ECG Findings
- Sgarbossa Criteria for STEMI Detection

11. Combination Blocks
- Definition and Clinical Context
- Diagnostic Approach
- Management Strategies

12. Junctional Rhythm
- Overview and ECG Characteristics
- Clinical Significance
- Treatment Considerations

13. Brugada Syndrome
- Definition and ECG Features
- Clinical Presentation
- Distinction Between Brugada Pattern and Syndrome
- Risk Stratification and Management
- Associated Channelopathies

14. Controversies in Management

- Evidence for Second-Line Antiarrhythmics
- Debates on Observation vs. Active Management

Chapter 5: Pulmonary Embolism

1. Introduction
    - Prevalence and mortality of pulmonary embolism (PE)
    - Challenges in diagnosis and management
    - Diagnostic guidelines
    - Anticoagulation therapy and advanced interventions
    - Prognostic tools and patient disposition

2. Aetiology, Pathogenesis, and Pathology
    - Risk factors for PE and Virchow's triad
    - Common causes of secondary PE
    - Impact of age and comorbidities on PE incidence
    - Hypercoagulable states and other contributing factors

3. Prevention
   - Preventive strategies for surgery and venous stasis
   - Thromboprophylaxis in high-risk patients
   - Early risk assessments for effective prevention

4. Clinical Features
   - History: Identifying key symptoms of PE
   - Physical examination findings and their diagnostic value
   - Risk factors and clinical presentation of PE

5. Risk Assessment for the Diagnosis of Pulmonary Embolism
   - Pre-test probability assessment using Wells and PERC scores
   - Utilization of D-dimer and imaging in risk stratification
   - Approach to anticoagulation before diagnosis

6. Imaging

- Role of chest X-ray in initial evaluation
- CT Pulmonary Angiography (CTPA) and its diagnostic accuracy
- Ventilation/Perfusion (V/Q) scanning: Indications and limitations
- Advances in V/Q SPECT (Single-Photon Emission Computed Tomography

7. Electrocardiography
    - Common ECG findings in PE and their clinical significance
    - Limitations of ECG in diagnosing PE

8. Pulmonary Embolism Diagnosis and Management
    - Detailed diagnostic strategies for PE
    - Imaging modalities: CTPA, V/Q scanning, and V/Q SPECT
    - Management of massive and submassive PE
    - Anticoagulation therapy and thrombolytic interventions

9. Prognosis and Risk Stratification

- Tools for assessing PE severity: SPESI, BNP, and troponin levels
- Clinical decision-making based on risk assessment and patient status

Chapter 6: Pericarditis, Cardiac Tamponade, and Myocarditis

1. Introduction
   - Overview of pericarditis and its types
   - Common association with "epi myocarditis" and its impact on diagnosis.
   - Causes of pericarditis and their clinical significance.

2. Clinical Features
   - History
   - Examination
   - High-Risk Features

3. Clinical Investigations
   - Blood Tests
   - Chest X-ray

- Electrocardiogram (ECG)
- Echocardiography
- Advanced Imaging
- Pericardiocentesis and Biopsy

4. Diagnosis
   - ESC Guidelines
   - Differentiating from Other Conditions

5. Classification of Pericarditis
   - Acute
   - Incessant
   - Chronic
   - Understanding the clinical course and classification based on symptoms duration.

6. Clinical Management and Treatment
   - General Approach
   - Non-Steroidal Anti-Inflammatory Drugs (NSAIDs)
   - Colchicine: Role in reducing recurrence and treatment regimen.

- Corticosteroids: Indications for second-line use, with cautions.
- Management in Pregnancy: Preferred treatments and contraindications during pregnancy.

7. Cardiac Tamponade: Non-Traumatic Case Management
    - Clinical Features
    - Investigations
    - Treatment: Mainstay of treatment, including pericardiocentesis and the management of underlying causes

Chapter 7: Heart Valve Emergencies: Overview and Clinical Management

1. Introduction
    - Overview of Heart Valve Emergencies
    - Significance and Impact on Cardiac Function

2. Infective Endocarditis: A Frequently Overlooked Diagnosis

- Importance of Early Diagnosis
- Epidemiology of Infective Endocarditis
- Risk Factors and Predisposing Conditions
- Pathophysiology of Infective Endocarditis
- Changing Microbial Landscape in Infective Endocarditis

3. Prevention and Prophylaxis

- Prophylactic Antibiotic Administration
- Guidelines for High-Risk Patients
- Recommended Prophylaxis for Various Procedures

4. Clinical Features of Infective Endocarditis

- Common Signs and Symptoms
- Systemic Embolization and Organ Involvement
- Clinical Examination Findings

5. Complications of Infective Endocarditis

- Cardiac Complications
- Neurological Complications

- Systemic Embolization
- Renal Dysfunction and Other Organ Involvement

6. Clinical Presentation and Diagnosis
   - Key Clinical Indicators
   - Diagnostic Investigations
   - Blood Cultures
   - Full Blood Count and Inflammatory Markers
   - Urinalysis
   - Echocardiography
   - Duke Criteria for Diagnosis

7. Treatment of Infective Endocarditis
   - Antibiotic Therapy and Empirical Treatment
   - Surgical Intervention Options
   - Role of Anticoagulation

8. Prognosis of Infective Endocarditis
   - Mortality and Morbidity Rates
   - Factors Affecting Prognosis
   - Long-Term Outcomes

9. Acute Aortic Incompetence
   - Etiology and Pathophysiology
   - Clinical Features and Management
   - Immediate Treatment Strategies

10. Mitral Stenosis: Acute Deterioration and Management
   - Pathophysiology of Mitral Stenosis
   - Acute Deterioration Triggers
   - Increased Heart Rate
   - Increased Flow Across the Stenosed Valve
   - Management and Treatment of Acute Deterioration

Chapter 8: Peripheral Vascular Disease

1. Arterial Disease
   - Classification of Ischaemia
   - Chronic Arterial Ischaemia
   - Epidemiology and pathogenesis
   - Clinical features of claudication and rest pain
   - Clinical investigations

- Treatment

2. Acute Arterial Ischaemia of the Lower Limb
    - Pathogenesis and causes
    - Clinical features and "6 Ps"
    - Differential diagnosis: Embolism vs. thrombosis
    - Treatment

3. Venous Disease and Deep Vein Thrombosis
    - DVT Diagnosis and Management
    - Diagnostic approach using ultrasound
    - Anticoagulation and treatment strategies
    - Graduated compression stockings and thrombolysis
    - Considerations for pregnant women and subclavian/axillary DVT
    - Direct factor Xa inhibitors as alternatives to traditional anticoagulants
    - Risk of post-thrombotic syndrome and thrombolytic therapy

4. Future Directions
    - Statin therapy in secondary prevention

- Impact of new anticoagulant therapies
- The role of emergency physicians in DVT diagnosis

5. Controversies
    - Evolving role of thrombolysis for arterial occlusion
    - Management of below-knee DVT, especially in pregnant women

Chapter 9: Hypertension

1. Introduction
    - Overview and Definition of Hypertension
    - Hypertensive Crises
    - Impact of Chronic Hypertension on Blood Pressure Tolerance
    - Advances in Treatment of Hypertensive Emergencies

2. Hypertensive Emergencies vs. Hypertensive Urgencies
    - Differentiating Emergencies from Urgencies

- Management of Hypertensive Emergencies
- Treatment of Hypertensive Urgencies

3. Epidemiology
   - Global Prevalence and Risk Factors
   - Disparities in Hypertension Rates
   - Diagnosis and Control Challenges

4. Hypertensive Emergencies
   - Neurological Hypertensive Emergencies
   - Hypertensive Encephalopathy
   - Stroke-Related Hypertension
   - Cardiovascular Hypertensive Emergencies
   - Acute Pulmonary Edema
   - Acute Coronary Syndrome
   - Acute Aortic Dissection
   - Renal Hypertensive Emergencies
   - Hypertensive Emergencies in Pregnancy

5. Clinical Evaluation of Hypertensive Crisis
   - Blood Pressure Measurement and Cardiovascular Examination
   - Neurological Evaluation

- Key Investigations: ECG, Urinalysis, Blood Tests, Imaging

6. Treatment

Goals of Treatment in Hypertensive Emergencies
- Parenteral Antihypertensive Agents
- MAP Reduction Targets
- Case-Specific Treatment Adjustments

7. Hypertensive Urgency: Evaluation and Treatment
- Approach to Asymptomatic Patients with Elevated BP
- Treatment Strategies: Gradual BP Reduction
- Use of ACE Inhibitors and Other First-Line Medications
- Follow-Up Care and Disposition

8. Prognosis and Disposition
- Prognosis Based on Effective Treatment
- Hospitalization vs. Outpatient Follow-Up

- Role of Comorbidities in Prognosis

9. Future Developments
   - Long-Term Management and Research
   - Role of Home Automated BP Monitoring

10. Controversies
    - Acute Stroke and BP Management
    - First-Line Therapy in Hypertensive Emergencies

Chapter 10: Aortic Dissection

1. Introduction
   - Overview of Aortic Dissection
   - Acute Aortic Syndrome and Pathophysiology

2. Epidemiology, Pathophysiology, and Classification
   - Incidence and Demographics
   - Risk Factors
   - Mechanisms of Dissection
   - Classification Systems

- Acute vs. Chronic Dissection

3. Clinical Features
    - Pain and Symptomatology
    - Neurological and Cardiovascular Manifestations
    - Examination Findings

4. Clinical Investigations
    - Diagnostic Workup
    - Imaging Modalities
    - Biomarkers for Early Detection
    - Differential Diagnosis

5. Aortic Dissection Management
    - Initial Treatment Strategy
    - Pharmacological Control of Pulsatile Load
    - Management of Type A Aortic Dissection
    - Management of Type B Aortic Dissection
    - Role of Endoluminal Stenting

6. Prognosis and Long-term Care
    - Survival Rates and Mortality
    - Post-surgical Care and Monitoring

- Lifelong Management with Beta-Blockade
- Long-term Imaging and Follow-up

List of Abbreviations

ACLS – Advanced Cardiovascular Life Support

AMI – Acute Myocardial Infarction

AORTA – Aortic Occlusion and Resuscitation Therapy for Acute

ATLS – Advanced Trauma Life Support

BP – Blood Pressure

CABG – Coronary Artery Bypass Grafting

CPR – Cardiopulmonary Resuscitation

ECG/EKG – Electrocardiogram

HF – Heart Failure

ICU – Intensive Care Unit

IV – Intravenous

LV – Left Ventricle

MI – Myocardial Infarction

NSTEMI – Non-ST Elevation Myocardial Infarction

STEMI – ST Elevation Myocardial Infarction

TIA – Transient Ischemic Attack

V-fib – Ventricular Fibrillation

V-tach – Ventricular Tachycardia

Introduction to Cardiovascular Emergencies

Cardiovascular emergencies represent a critical area of healthcare, involving life-threatening conditions that require rapid diagnosis, intervention, and management. These emergencies encompass a broad spectrum of acute conditions affecting the heart and blood vessels, which, if not promptly addressed, can result in severe complications or death. The prevalence of cardiovascular disease, including acute coronary syndromes, aortic dissection, arrhythmias, heart failure, and pulmonary embolism, underscores the importance of understanding the mechanisms, clinical manifestations, and management strategies for these emergencies.

The emergency care of cardiovascular conditions demands a multifaceted approach, incorporating both immediate life-saving interventions and long-term therapeutic strategies to stabilize the patient and prevent further deterioration. A hallmark of effective cardiovascular emergency care is the ability to rapidly identify high-risk conditions, initiate appropriate therapies, and prioritize resources, particularly when patients present with unstable or critical symptoms.

For instance, acute coronary syndromes (ACS), including myocardial infarction, present with varying degrees of severity but often share common features such as chest pain, shortness of breath, and potentially fatal arrhythmias. Identifying ACS early and applying interventions like antiplatelet therapy, thrombolytics, or percutaneous coronary interventions (PCI) can significantly improve patient outcomes. Similarly, conditions like aortic dissection and hypertensive crises demand immediate recognition and management, often involving invasive measures to control hemodynamics and prevent life-threatening complications such as rupture.

Additionally, arrhythmias, whether supraventricular or ventricular, can lead to hemodynamic instability, requiring swift management to restore normal rhythm and prevent collapse or cardiac arrest. The role of advanced resuscitation techniques, including defibrillation and pharmacologic interventions, is central to the stabilization of patients with severe arrhythmias or cardiac arrest.

The timely recognition of these emergencies often requires advanced diagnostic tools, including electrocardiography (ECG), echocardiography, computed tomography (CT), and magnetic resonance imaging (MRI). Moreover, biomarkers, such as troponins and D-dimer, have gained interest in aiding the diagnosis and rule-out of certain conditions like myocardial infarction and aortic dissection. However, the limitations of these biomarkers in specific clinical contexts highlight the importance of integrating clinical judgment with diagnostic testing.

In this context, the management of cardiovascular emergencies revolves around a structured protocol that emphasizes rapid diagnosis, stabilization, and targeted therapy. For example, in patients presenting with aortic dissection, the primary goal is to control the heart rate and blood pressure, preventing the progression of the dissection and reducing the risk of rupture. In contrast, for myocardial infarction, early reperfusion therapies, such as thrombolysis or PCI, are critical in restoring blood flow to ischemic myocardial tissue.

Ultimately, the effective management of cardiovascular emergencies hinges on a comprehensive understanding of the pathophysiology, clinical presentation, diagnostic approaches, and therapeutic interventions for each condition. It also requires a collaborative effort among healthcare professionals, including emergency physicians, cardiologists, intensivists, and surgeons, to optimize patient outcomes. By providing a systematic approach to the evaluation and treatment of these acute conditions, healthcare providers can improve survival rates and minimize long-term complications, ultimately enhancing patient care in these high-stakes clinical scenarios.

Chapter 1
Chest Pain

Introduction

Chest pain is a frequent complaint encountered in emergency medicine and can be regarded as a prototypical emergency issue. While many causes are benign, the differential diagnoses include life-threatening conditions. Emergency providers must utilize a combination of thorough assessment, risk stratification tools, hospital-specific pathways, and clinical judgment to manage these patients effectively and safely.

Epidemiology

According to the Australian Institute for Health and Welfare's 2017 report, chest and throat pain ranked as the second most common primary diagnosis in emergency department (ED) visits, following abdominal and pelvic pain. This category accounted for 3.6% of all ED presentations, as per the ICD-10-AM classification. Furthermore, ischemic heart disease remains the leading cause of death in Western nations.

The incidence of acute chest pain in the ED appears to be on the rise, with public health campaigns increasing awareness of the need for immediate treatment of myocardial infarction (MI), leading to more frequent ED visits for chest pain. Additionally, emergency ambulance responses have largely replaced general practitioners for these patients. Interestingly, while the incidence of coronary heart disease is decreasing in developed countries, patients presenting with chest pain are showing a declining prevalence of acute coronary syndromes (ACS) and an increasing incidence of less severe conditions.

Differential Diagnosis and Approach

The differential diagnosis for acute chest pain includes conditions that range from benign to life-threatening. Acute coronary syndrome (ACS), which includes unstable angina (UA), ST-elevation myocardial infarction (STEMI), and non-ST-elevation myocardial infarction (NSTEMI), is the primary concern, being both common and potentially fatal. Other serious conditions like pulmonary embolism (PE) and aortic dissection must also be considered in patients presenting with chest pain, which may radiate to the jaw, shoulders, or upper abdomen.

Historical distinctions between "typical" and "atypical" chest pain are less useful in diagnosis, particularly in older patients. All patients should be assessed based on their clinical presentation and risk profile, without solely relying on traditional cardiac risk factors. While risk factors identified by studies such as the Framingham Heart Study are valuable on a population level, they offer limited diagnostic utility in individual cases of chest pain.

Musculoskeletal causes of chest pain, such as Tietze syndrome (costochondritis), epidemic myalgia (Bornholm disease), and herpes zoster, may present with pain that can be mistaken for more serious conditions. Gastro-oesophageal reflux disease (GERD), esophageal spasms, and peptic ulcer disease can also mimic MI pain, especially if the discomfort is related to food intake or position changes.

Other potential causes of chest pain include spontaneous pneumothorax, pericarditis (often viral), pleurisy (commonly secondary to respiratory infections or PE), and abdominal conditions such as biliary colic, pancreatitis, or peptic ulcers. Anxiety can contribute to chest pain but is rarely the sole cause. A considerable number of patients may ultimately be diagnosed with "non-specific chest pain" after ED evaluation.

Clinical Features

The primary goal of clinical assessment is to identify patients with a high risk of serious pathology who require further investigation or inpatient care. The risk stratification process often focuses on identifying those at risk for ACS, given its high prevalence and potential severity.

ACS typically presents with chest pain described as crushing, gripping, or squeezing, and may radiate to the left arm. However, distinguishing between "typical" and "atypical" presentations of ACS is not particularly helpful, especially in older patients. Clinical predictors, such as pain radiating to both shoulders or diaphoresis, can help in identifying ACS. While coronary heart disease risk factors are important, they provide limited diagnostic value in individual cases of chest pain.

Clinical examination can help identify non-cardiac causes of chest pain, such as musculoskeletal tenderness or complications from ACS, like arrhythmias, heart failure, or cardiogenic shock. Reproducible chest wall tenderness is not suggestive of ACS but does not rule it out completely.

PE is suspected in cases of pleuritic chest pain associated with breathlessness or a history of risk factors such as deep vein thrombosis, immobilization, recent trauma, or malignancy. Clinical examination may reveal tachycardia or features of deep vein thrombosis. When PE is suspected, evidence-based decision algorithms, such as the Wells criteria and PERC rule, should be employed.

Aortic dissection typically presents with severe chest pain radiating to the back, along with diaphoresis, syncope, or neurological symptoms. Clinical findings, such as blood pressure discrepancies between the arms or pulse delays, should raise suspicion. The likelihood of aortic dissection increases with the number of clinical findings.

In cases of chest pain, a thorough abdominal examination is crucial to identify conditions like biliary colic, cholecystitis, or pancreatitis, which can manifest as chest pain.

Clinical Investigations

The electrocardiogram (ECG) is a vital diagnostic tool for all patients presenting with acute, non-traumatic chest pain. A normal ECG does not exclude a myocardial infarction, but specific changes such as ST-segment elevation, new Q waves, or conduction defects are highly suggestive of acute MI. In PE, ECG changes may include sinus tachycardia, signs of acute pulmonary hypertension, or the McGinn-White sign (S1Q3T3 pattern).

While the ECG has limited sensitivity and specificity for aortic dissection, changes in the right coronary artery ostia may suggest inferior ischemia. Repeating the ECG is essential, especially when clinical suspicion persists or when the patient initially presents with chest pain but later becomes asymptomatic.

Chest radiographs are often used in the assessment of patients with chest pain, primarily to identify non-cardiac causes such as pneumothorax or rib fractures, as well as complications from myocardial infarction (MI) like left ventricular failure. Despite being frequently ordered, chest x-rays are usually not helpful in the diagnosis.

The measurement of serum troponin levels plays a crucial role in both evidence-based risk stratification for acute coronary syndromes (ACS) and in preventing unnecessary practices that could lead to unnecessary admissions or harm. With the high sensitivity of modern troponin assays for detecting myocardial damage, it is essential to use these tests judiciously.

High-sensitivity troponin (hsT) assays, recommended by both the National Heart Foundation and the European Society of Cardiology, are now commonly employed in emergency departments. The third universal definition of MI specifies that hsT assays can detect circulating troponin in most healthy individuals, offering accurate reference ranges and demonstrating acceptable imprecision at the 99th percentile. Compared to older, less sensitive tests, hsT assays can detect MI earlier, require fewer repeat tests, and have greater sensitivity for detecting smaller cardiac events. However, they also carry a risk of false-positive results, leading to unnecessary hospital admissions and patient anxiety due to their reduced specificity. While elevated troponin levels can indicate myocardial injury, they may not always be clinically significant, as seen in long-distance runners.

It is important to recognize that troponin elevation is not exclusive to MI, and low troponin levels may not necessarily indicate significant heart pathology. Elevated troponin levels can also be seen in conditions such as pulmonary embolism, sepsis, renal failure, burns, and heart failure, among others.

If ACS is suspected, repeat troponin testing is advised when initial levels are inconclusive or below the reference range within a defined time frame. The National Heart Foundation and the Cardiac Society of Australia and New Zealand recommend repeat hsT testing at 2 hours for patients with a low Thrombolysis in Myocardial Infarction (TIMI) score and at 6 hours for those with higher scores, or at 12 hours when using traditional troponin assays.

Local guidelines on troponin testing vary, so it is important to consult institutional protocols, as these may reflect assay performance or patient population characteristics. Many emergency departments have chest pain units for the observation, serial testing, and management of such patients. These units often combine serial troponin testing with functional or anatomical cardiac tests, including exercise ECG, coronary CT angiography (CTCA), and calcium scoring, which primarily assess the long-term risk in asymptomatic individuals.

Further cardiac testing, such as exercise ECG or myocardial perfusion studies, may be appropriate for non-low-risk patients suspected of having ACS. Guidelines from various international societies advocate for such testing, though there is some disagreement on the timing, with most recommending it during hospitalization or soon after discharge. It is crucial to follow local protocols or develop them in collaboration with relevant stakeholders.

Various clinical risk scores, such as the TIMI, HEART (History, ECG, Age, Risk factors, Troponin), and EDACS (Emergency Department Assessment of Chest Pain), are used to help stratify the risk for ACS in emergency department patients. While these tools can provide useful information, they should complement the overall patient evaluation, not replace it. Some scores, like the HEART score, have shown better performance in predicting major adverse cardiac events compared to other tools, such as TIMI or GRACE scores.

Guidelines from the National Heart Foundation and the Cardiac Society of Australia and New Zealand strongly recommend using evidence-based protocols for suspected ACS that include formal risk stratification. These protocols are crucial for guiding patient management and ensuring the appropriate level of care.

In populations such as Aboriginal and Torres Strait Islander peoples, or those with HIV, clinicians should maintain a higher index of suspicion for coronary disease, although these factors are not typically considered in standard risk stratification tools.

The diagnostic approach to other conditions like pulmonary embolism (PE) and thoracic aortic dissection also requires careful attention. For PE, a D-dimer test may be appropriate in low-risk patients with a negative Wells score, while advanced imaging is needed for higher-risk individuals. In the case of thoracic aortic dissection, a chest x-ray may reveal signs like a widened mediastinum, but a CT angiogram (CTA) is typically required for confirmation.

The treatment of chest pain is tailored to the underlying cause, with specific chapters dedicated to the management of ACS, pulmonary embolism, and aortic dissection. In the case of suspected ACS, early treatment with aspirin, oxygen, and, if needed, nitroglycerin or morphine is recommended while awaiting a definitive diagnosis. Musculoskeletal chest pain should be managed with analgesics, while gastro-oesophageal pain can be treated with antacids or proton pump inhibitors. Anxiety should also be considered as a contributing factor, and patients should be encouraged to follow up for counseling or treatment if necessary.

For patients with non-specific chest pain, the prognosis is generally good, with many experiencing no further episodes in the following month. This period also offers an opportunity to address cardiac risk factors, particularly smoking, and to provide general advice on diet and exercise. Patients with abnormal findings in blood pressure, glucose, or lipid levels should be referred to their general practitioner for further evaluation and long-term management.

Disposition decisions should be based on the severity of the condition and the patient's access to follow-up care. High-risk patients, even those with negative tests, should be admitted for further observation. Using flowcharts, such as those developed by the National Heart Foundation of Australia, can help guide disposition and additional testing.

The prognosis of chest pain patients largely depends on the underlying cause, with those without a clear diagnosis after clinical assessment, ECG, and troponin testing typically having an excellent outlook. However, even when cardiac disease is ruled out, these patients still have a higher risk of future cardiac events compared to the general population.

References

1. Dezman ZD, Mattu A, Body R. The role of history and physical examination in diagnosing acute coronary syndromes in emergency department patients. West J Emerg Med. 2017;18(4):752-760. https://doi.org/10.5811/westjem.2017.3.32666.

2. Goodacre S, Thokala P, Carroll C, et al. A systematic review, meta-analysis, and economic modeling of diagnostic strategies for suspected acute coronary syndrome. Health Technol Assess. 2013;17(1):v-vi, 1-188.

https://www.ncbi.nlm.nih.gov/pubmed/23331845.

3. Hulten EA, Carbonaro S, Petrillo SP, et al. Prognostic significance of cardiac computed tomography angiography: a systematic review and meta-analysis. J Am Coll Cardiol. 2011;57(10):1237-1247.

4. National Heart Foundation. Clinical Guidelines for the Management of Acute Coronary Syndromes. 2016.

5. NICE Guidelines. Acute Coronary Syndrome Guidelines.

6. Poldervaart JM, Langedijk M, Backus BE, et al. Comparison of the GRACE, HEART, and TIMI scores in predicting major adverse cardiac events in chest pain patients in the emergency department. Int J Cardiol. 2017;227:656-661.

7. Webster R, Norman P, Goodacre S, Thompson A. Psychological outcomes in patients with acute non-cardiac chest pain: a systematic review. Emerg Med J. 2012;29(4):267-273.

Chapter 2
Acute Coronary Syndromes
Rohan Laging

Essentials

1. A 12-lead ECG should be performed and interpreted within 10 minutes of a patient's arrival to assess potential acute coronary syndrome (ACS) and determine the need for reperfusion therapy.

2. Aspirin should be administered to all patients with suspected ACS unless contraindicated.

3. The ECG alone cannot rule out ACS.

4. Risk stratification should be carried out for all patients presenting with possible ACS, and management should be guided by a suspected ACS assessment protocol (suspected ACS-AP).

5. For patients with ST-elevation myocardial infarction (STEMI), percutaneous coronary intervention (PCI) is preferred over thrombolysis for reperfusion, provided it can be performed within 90 minutes.

6. In STEMI cases, emergency clinicians must act quickly and decisively to initiate reperfusion therapy.

7. Primary prevention of ACS requires a comprehensive cardiovascular risk assessment, which is best conducted in primary care settings.

Introduction to Acute Coronary Syndrome (ACS)

Acute coronary syndrome (ACS) is one of the most common and critical conditions encountered in emergency medicine. Prompt recognition and treatment are essential to minimize preventable morbidity and mortality.

ACS includes a range of related conditions, such as ST-elevation myocardial infarction (STEMI), non-ST-elevation myocardial infarction (NSTEMI), and non-ST-elevation acute coronary syndrome (NSTEACS), which encompasses both NSTEMI and unstable angina (UA). In some cases, the presence of a new left bundle branch block (LBBB) alongside an acute myocardial infarction (AMI) is treated as STEMI, since it follows the same management approach. AMI is defined by the death of heart muscle cells due to prolonged lack of blood supply (ischemia).

Recent advances in diagnostics, especially with high-sensitivity biomarkers, have expanded the diagnostic criteria for ACS, making it essential for clinicians to stay updated on the latest definitions and diagnostic strategies.

For a more in-depth understanding of the diagnostic process and risk assessment for ACS.

Patients presenting with suspected ACS should undergo formal risk assessment to guide their management. This is typically done using structured protocols that combine validated risk scores, such as the TIMI or HEART scores, alongside electrocardiogram (ECG) findings and biomarker levels. These protocols help determine the appropriate treatment and whether the patient can be safely discharged or requires further investigation.

For example, protocols like the ADAPT (2-hour accelerated diagnostic protocol) have shown to be highly effective in identifying patients who are at very low risk for major adverse cardiac events (MACE), with a negative predictive value greater than 99%. Such tools are invaluable in enabling early discharge for patients who do not require prolonged hospitalization, thus reducing unnecessary healthcare costs. Emergency departments should collaborate with cardiologists and laboratory teams to develop and refine their ACS management protocols.

Well-established risk factors for ischemic heart disease (IHD), such as those identified in the Framingham study, are widely recognized by clinicians and patients. These factors—like age, family history, hypertension, and smoking—play a key role in risk stratification for ACS. Additionally, emerging research continues to highlight the importance of other factors, such as diabetes and lipid profiles, in refining risk assessment and improving patient outcomes.

The relationship between Human Immunodeficiency Virus (HIV) and Ischemic Heart Disease (IHD) should be explored when assessing patients presenting with possible Acute Coronary Syndrome (ACS), as this is an important consideration in the clinical evaluation.

Pathophysiology

ACS is primarily caused by the disruption of the coronary artery's endothelial lining, leading to the formation of a thrombus that obstructs blood flow, resulting in myocardial ischemia or infarction. The severity of the infarction depends on factors such as the duration and extent of the blockage, myocardial oxygen demand, and underlying physiological conditions like anemia and circulating catecholamines.

Patients may be asymptomatic despite having coronary atheromas, especially when the atheromas are not large enough to obstruct blood flow. However, when the atheromas rupture, leading to sudden vessel occlusion, a myocardial infarction (MI) may occur. The classic symptoms of an MI include severe, crushing chest pain, often associated with a rapid onset of symptoms. Chest pain that is reproducible with palpation and occurs in a pleuritic pattern is less likely to indicate ACS and may suggest other diagnoses.

ACS is not solely the result of atherosclerotic blockages. Conditions such as Prinzmetal angina, which is caused by coronary artery spasm, can also lead to myocardial ischemia and may present with transient ST-segment elevation on an ECG. Coronary angiography in such cases may show minor atheromas or normal coronary vessels. Rare causes of coronary occlusion include Kawasaki disease, aortic dissection involving the coronary artery ostia, and spontaneous coronary artery dissection.

The clinical presentation and complications of ACS largely depend on the location of the coronary artery occlusion. The most common location for myocardial infarction is the anterior or antero-septal region, typically due to occlusion of the Left Anterior Descending (LAD) artery, and it is associated with a worse prognosis. Other infarctions include lateral (circumflex artery or diagonal branch of the LAD), inferior (Right Coronary Artery (RCA) or circumflex), and posterior infarctions (typically from RCA or circumflex artery in cases of left coronary dominance). Complications, such as right ventricular failure, can occur in inferior and posterior infarctions.

Epidemiology

While coronary heart disease (CHD) mortality has decreased in Western countries over the past several decades, it remains a leading cause of death, accounting for approximately one-third of all fatalities in individuals over 35 years of age. In the United States, nearly half of middle-aged men and a third of middle-aged women will experience some form of CHD.

In Australia, the age-standardized rate of acute coronary events is significantly higher in men than in women. The rate of acute coronary events rises with age, with those over 85 years experiencing a rate more than three times higher than those aged 65–74 years. Over the period from 2007 to 2012, the rate of acute coronary events in Australia declined by 24%.

Clinical Features

A detailed clinical assessment is essential in suspected ACS cases. The presence of chest pain radiating to the right or both shoulders, sweating, shortness of breath, vomiting, or a previous MI is strongly suggestive of ACS. On the other hand, pleuritic pain or pain that is reproducible on palpation is less likely to indicate ACS.

The distinction between stable angina and ACS is vital. Stable angina is characterized by predictable pain triggered by exertion, which is relieved by rest or glyceryl trinitrate (GTN). Unstable Angina (UA), a form of ACS, presents with more severe, unpredictable pain that occurs with less exertion and may increase in frequency or intensity.

Physical examination is generally not helpful in diagnosing ACS but is crucial for identifying complications such as heart failure. Signs of heart failure may include poor peripheral circulation, tachycardia, pulmonary crackles, and elevated jugular venous pressure.

Diagnosis

The most important diagnostic tool for ACS is the 12-lead ECG, which should be performed and interpreted by an experienced clinician within 10 minutes of a patient's arrival. If the initial ECG is unclear, it should be repeated as the clinical situation evolves. For example, an ECG performed after pain relief can help diagnose Wellen syndrome, which indicates critical stenosis of the left anterior descending artery.

In STEMI diagnosis, key criteria include:

Persistent (>20 minutes) ST-elevation in two or more contiguous leads.

The presence of new onset Left Bundle Branch Block (LBBB), which can be challenging to diagnose, especially without prior ECGs.

The Sgarbossa criteria can assist in diagnosing STEMI in patients with a prior LBBB. These criteria involve evaluating the ST elevation in concordance with the QRS complex and other related criteria.

The location of ischemic changes on an ECG helps pinpoint the affected coronary vessel:

LAD: Anteroseptal changes.

Left Circumflex (LCx): Anterolateral changes.

RCA: Inferior changes.

Posterior descending artery (PDA): Posterior changes.

Management of NSTE ACS Patients

In patients with Non-ST Elevation Acute Coronary Syndromes (NSTEACS), there is a reduction in recurrent myocardial infarction (MI) and cardiovascular re-hospitalization within 12 months, but mortality benefits are likely absent. Regardless, all NSTE ACS patients should receive urgent cardiology consultation in the emergency department (ED). Initiating therapy promptly requires adherence to a clinical pathway, collaboratively developed with pre-hospital services, emergency physicians, cardiologists, and clinical pharmacists. For centers with primary percutaneous coronary intervention (PCI) capabilities, the pathway should aim to minimize door-to-balloon (DTB) time to under 60 minutes. For centers without primary PCI, patients should be transferred to PCI-capable centers, ensuring the total time from first medical contact to balloon time does not exceed 90 minutes, or in case of unsuccessful thrombolysis, within 3 to 24 hours post-thrombolysis. Immediate transfer to a PCI center is required for all STEMI cases complicated by cardiogenic shock.

Thrombolysis and PCI Timing

For patients presenting more than 12 hours after initial symptoms, thrombolysis is contraindicated, and transfer to a PCI-capable center should be arranged promptly, though not as an emergency. This approach maximizes the potential benefit from PCI therapy.

Risk-Benefit Assessment for Bleeding Risk Therapies

When considering therapies that may increase bleeding risk, a personalized assessment of benefits and harms should be conducted. Expert cardiology input is crucial when initiating therapies that include:

P2Y12 Receptor Inhibitors

These drugs, which inhibit platelet function, are recommended in addition to aspirin for patients with confirmed ACS at intermediate or high risk of recurrent ischemic events, including STEMI cases. Ticagrelor (180 mg initially, then 90 mg twice daily) and prasugrel (60 mg initially, then

10 mg daily) have shown to reduce mortality and recurrent MI compared to clopidogrel (300–600 mg initially, then 75 mg daily). However, ticagrelor and prasugrel increase the risk of major bleeding, making clopidogrel a better option for older patients or those with lower body weight or a history of transient ischemic attacks or strokes.

Glycoprotein IIb/IIIa Inhibitors

These drugs, used alongside heparin, are initiated in ACS patients undergoing or preparing for PCI, particularly those with high-risk angiographic features or thrombotic complications. They are not routinely initiated in the ED. Agents in this class include abciximab, tirofiban, and eptifibatide.

Antithrombin Therapy

For ACS patients at intermediate to very high risk of ischemic events, enoxaparin or unfractionated heparin (UFH) is recommended.

Enoxaparin inhibits factor Xa and is dosed subcutaneously twice daily, whereas UFH potentiates antithrombin III to inactivate thrombin and factor Xa. Enoxaparin is preferred for its simpler dosing regimen and does not require activated partial thromboplastin time (aPTT) monitoring.

Direct Thrombin Inhibitors

Bivalirudin, an alternative to glycoprotein IIb/IIIa inhibitors and heparin, may reduce bleeding risks in ACS patients. The decision to use this therapy requires expert evaluation.

β-Blockers

β-blockers should be initiated non-urgently, unless contraindicated, to reduce myocardial oxygen demand and improve outcomes in ACS patients.

Patient Disposition

Patients with ACS should be admitted to a coronary care unit (CCU), with the possibility of transferring to the cardiac catheterization laboratory before CCU depending on the severity of the ACS. Patients post-emergent coronary artery bypass grafting (CABG), with cardiogenic shock, or severe acute medical comorbidities may require intensive care unit (ICU) care.

Common Complications in ACS

Arrhythmias and Conduction Disturbances

Arrhythmias are common in ACS and can range from benign to life-threatening. Management strategies should address underlying ischemia and rhythm disturbances promptly.

Pericarditis

Pericarditis, often occurring post-MI, requires differentiation from other causes of chest pain.

Treatment typically involves anti-inflammatory medications.

Acute Left Ventricular Failure and Cardiogenic Shock

Left ventricular failure is a common complication of MI and can vary in severity. Management includes optimizing oxygenation, correcting electrolyte imbalances, and using inotropes when necessary. PCI can improve outcomes for STEMI patients with cardiogenic shock, while LV assist devices may be used in select patients.

Thromboembolism

Thromboembolism, resulting from thrombus formation on hypokinetic myocardium, is a risk in large anterior infarctions, especially when LV aneurysm is present. Anticoagulation therapy is used to reduce the risk of embolic events.

Mechanical Complications

Mechanical defects such as ventricular aneurysm formation, acute mitral insufficiency, ventricular septal defects, and free wall rupture can occur. These require immediate surgical intervention.

Complications of Therapy

Major bleeding, particularly intracerebral hemorrhage, is a known risk with antiplatelet and anticoagulation therapies. Balancing the risk of bleeding with therapeutic benefit is crucial, and shared decision-making with patients or their representatives is often necessary. PCI-related complications include coronary artery perforation, radial or femoral entry site issues, and stent-related thrombosis.

Prognosis

Prognosis in ACS patients depends on multiple factors, including age, comorbidities, the extent of coronary disease, LV dysfunction, mechanical complications, and arrhythmias. Initial treatment response also plays a significant role in long-term outcomes.

Primary and Secondary Prevention

Patients presenting with ACS should be encouraged to engage in lifestyle modifications to reduce their risk factors for ischemic heart disease (IHD). Discharged patients should be prescribed a combination of medications, including aspirin, a P2Y12 inhibitor, statins, vasodilatory beta-blockers (if EF ≤40%), and ACE inhibitors or angiotensin receptor blockers if indicated. Referral to cardiac rehabilitation is also recommended.

Controversies in ACS Management

There are ongoing debates surrounding the optimal use of ultra-short suspected ACS protocols, the role of coronary artery CT and calcium scores in chest pain evaluation, and the definition of specific patient groups for further investigation with provocative tests.

Determining which patients require cardiac monitoring, both in the ED and during hospitalization, remains a topic of clinical research and guideline refinement.

Chapter 3
Acute Pulmonary Oedema (APO)

Essentials

1. High Morbidity and Mortality: Severe acute pulmonary oedema (APO) is linked to significant morbidity and mortality, making timely and effective intervention critical.

2. Pathophysiological Features: APO is primarily characterized by an abnormal distribution of fluid in the lungs. It is important to note that fluid overload is not present in the majority of patients with APO.

3. Diagnostic Approach: The diagnosis of APO is based on a comprehensive clinical evaluation, including a detailed patient history, focused physical examination, and diagnostic tests such as ECG, lung ultrasound, and chest X-ray.

4. Therapeutic Goals: Management focuses on ensuring adequate oxygenation and maintaining cardiac output while addressing the underlying causes of the condition. Identifying and correcting any reversible etiologies is a key aspect of treatment.

5. Management of Hypotension: Patients experiencing hypotension should receive both ventilatory support and inotropic therapy to stabilize their condition.

6. Standard Therapeutic Interventions: The primary treatments for APO include oxygen therapy, vasodilation (typically with nitrates), and non-invasive ventilation (NIV).

7. Effectiveness of NIV: Non-invasive ventilation has proven to be both safe and effective in managing APO. It has been shown to reduce the need for intubation, decrease the likelihood of ICU admission, and improve overall survival rates.

Assessment and Management of Acute Pulmonary Oedema

Effective management of acute pulmonary oedema necessitates rapid assessment and the implementation of appropriate therapies tailored to the patient's condition, including the management of oxygenation, fluid balance, and underlying pathophysiology.

Introduction

Acute Pulmonary Oedema (APO) primarily affects elderly individuals and is associated with poor long-term outcomes, especially when severe. It is a pathological condition characterized by fluid accumulation in the alveolar spaces, leading to impaired gas exchange and reduced lung compliance. The resulting symptoms include acute dyspnoea, hypoxia, and increased respiratory effort. APO occurs when factors such as increased pulmonary capillary pressure, reduced plasma oncotic pressure, or changes in capillary permeability cause fluid leakage from capillaries into the pulmonary interstitium. When the rate of fluid accumulation exceeds the ability of lymphatic drainage, alveolar flooding occurs.

Aetiology and Pathophysiology

The causes of APO are categorized into cardiogenic and noncardiogenic types. Cardiogenic APO, the most common cause in emergency departments, arises from an acute decrease in cardiac output due to left atrial outflow obstruction or left ventricular (LV) dysfunction, compounded by increased systemic vascular resistance (SVR). This results in backpressure on the pulmonary vasculature and elevated pulmonary capillary pressure. Over time, this leads to a vicious cycle: worsening oxygenation and increasing pulmonary vascular resistance, which aggravates LV dysfunction and pulmonary oedema. Often, patients experience fluid maldistribution rather than true fluid overload, which has shifted management strategies from high-dose diuretics to the use of vasodilators and non-invasive ventilation (NIV) to improve cardiac output by reducing SVR.

In non-cardiogenic APO, increased pulmonary vascular permeability due to various insults leads to fluid leakage into the alveolar spaces. This type may also result from damage to alveolar cells, impairing their ability to clear oedema fluid.

Clinical Assessment

History

Clinical assessment and management should proceed simultaneously in an emergency setting. Typically, patients present with sudden-onset severe dyspnoea, which may be described as a sensation of drowning. A focused history should include questions about recent chest pain, palpitations, a history of ischaemic heart disease, worsening congestive heart failure, or other underlying causes. Current medications and adherence should also be explored.

Examination

On examination, patients often appear pale or cyanotic, sweating profusely and anxious. If hypoxic or hypercapnic, they may display confusion. They often maintain an upright posture to ease breathing and may be unable to sit still. Pink or white frothy sputum may be expectorated, contributing to the feeling of drowning. Tachycardia, increased respiratory rate, and the use of accessory muscles for breathing are common signs. Hypoxia is evident with low oxygen saturations. Most patients will be hypertensive or normotensive, while hypotension indicates cardiogenic shock and carries a poor prognosis. Skin mottling and signs of poor peripheral perfusion suggest worsening cardiac function. Elevated jugular venous pressure (JVP), a third heart sound, or gallop rhythm are indicative of cardiogenic APO, but these signs are absent in non-cardiogenic cases.

The chest may be dull to percussion, with fine crepitations heard upon auscultation, typically starting at the lung bases but potentially progressing as oedema worsens. Adventitious lung sounds like wheeze or "cardiac asthma" may also be present.

Clinical Investigations

Electrocardiogram (ECG)

An ECG is crucial for detecting acute ischaemia or arrhythmias. If ST-elevation myocardial infarction (STEMI) is identified, immediate reperfusion strategies should be employed.

Imaging

A chest X-ray typically reveals an enlarged heart and can distinguish APO from other conditions like airway diseases. Initial findings may show prominent upper-lobe veins, with worsening oedema leading to interstitial changes like Kerley B lines, indicating basilar and hilar infiltrates. In severe APO, alveolar oedema becomes evident, and pleural effusions may develop if interstitial pressure exceeds pleural pressure. These imaging findings may also reflect the underlying cause, such as cardiomegaly in cardiogenic APO.

Ultrasound (US) is increasingly used in the emergency department, with high sensitivity and specificity for diagnosing APO. Vertical comet tail artifacts (B lines) originating from the pleural line indicate pulmonary oedema. In more severe cases, B lines extend upwards. The US can help differentiate causes of dyspnoea, such as acute respiratory distress syndrome (ARDS), acute lung injury, or airways disease.

Blood Tests

Blood tests should assess:

Hemoglobin: to rule out anemia as a cause.

Electrolytes: to identify abnormalities caused by diuretics, ACE inhibitors, or renal failure.

Cardiac biomarkers: to assess for myocardial injury, or specific tests like lipase for suspected pancreatitis.

Blood gasses: to identify acid-base imbalances and guide treatment.

Natriuretic peptides: BNP or NT-proBNP can help distinguish APO from other causes of acute dyspnoea. Elevated levels (>500 pg/mL for BNP or age-specific cutoffs for NT-proBNP) strongly suggest acute heart failure, while low levels make it less likely.

Oximetry

Oximetry, sometimes supplemented by blood gasses, can help monitor severity and track the patient's response to treatment. In severe cases, invasive monitoring may be necessary.

Treatment

Management should focus on providing supportive care to optimize cardiac output and oxygenation, followed by treatment of the underlying cause.

Non-cardiogenic Pulmonary Oedema

In non-cardiogenic APO, the primary approach involves removing the patient from the causative environment, supporting oxygenation through non-invasive or invasive ventilation, and treating the underlying cause. In cases of lung injury, low-volume, low-pressure, lung-protective ventilation is recommended.

Cardiogenic Pulmonary Oedema

The majority of APO cases in the emergency department are cardiogenic. Treatment strategies are based on the patient's haemodynamic status:

1. Normotensive or Hypertensive Patients: Treatment should focus on reducing preload and afterload using nitrates and optimizing oxygenation, often with non-invasive ventilation. Patients should be kept in an upright position to reduce ventilation-perfusion mismatch and ease breathing.

2. Pharmacotherapy:

Nitrates: The cornerstone of pharmacological therapy for APO. Nitrates work by increasing cyclic GMP in vascular smooth muscle, leading to venodilation and a reduction in preload. This also helps counteract the effects of catecholamines released during an APO episode. At higher doses, nitrates also reduce afterload, improving cardiac output.

Morphine

Morphine was previously a common treatment for Acute Pulmonary Oedema (APO), as it induces vasodilation and reduces sympathetic activation. However, its use is associated with notable adverse effects, including respiratory depression, central nervous system suppression, hypotension, reduced cardiac output, and an increased risk of vomiting and aspiration. Studies, including small prospective trials and larger retrospective studies, have shown that morphine use in APO patients correlates with higher rates of intubation, ICU admissions, and mortality. Given the lack of evidence supporting its benefit and the emerging data linking it to harm, morphine is no longer recommended for managing APO.

Aspirin

In APO patients, myocardial ischaemia or infarction is a leading cause. Aspirin is effective in reducing the risk of death and subsequent myocardial infarctions in these cases. Although aspirin does not directly treat APO, it should be administered when myocardial ischaemia is suspected as the underlying cause.

Ventilatory Support

Patients with APO are typically hypoxic and require high-flow oxygen therapy to meet their respiratory demands. A system such as a Venturi mask can effectively deliver the necessary oxygen volume. If left untreated, hypoxia exacerbates APO by causing pulmonary vasoconstriction and reducing myocardial oxygen delivery. However, prolonged exposure to high oxygen levels should be avoided in patients with pre-existing chronic lung conditions. Oxygen should be administered conservatively, gradually reduced as the patient stabilizes, aiming for normal saturation levels.

Patients with altered consciousness, cardiogenic shock, respiratory failure, or respiratory arrest need endotracheal intubation with mechanical ventilation, ideally performed through rapid-sequence intubation. If pre-oxygenation is inadequate, delayed-sequence intubation may be necessary. Non-invasive ventilation (NIV) options such as Continuous Positive Airway Pressure (CPAP) or Bi-Level Positive Airway Pressure (BiPAP) are useful for patients who can avoid intubation. CPAP typically starts at pressures of 5–10 cm H2O, while BiPAP begins with expiratory pressures at 3–5 cm H2O and inspiratory pressures 5–8 cm H2O higher. These treatments improve oxygenation and ventilation by expanding alveoli, increasing gas exchange, and reducing the work of breathing.

CPAP and BiPAP have shown benefits over conventional treatment, improving oxygenation, ventilation, and heart rate, with reduced rates of intubation, ICU admissions, and mortality. BiPAP may be especially beneficial for patients with coexisting respiratory diseases or acute chronic respiratory acidosis, as it provides quicker symptom relief. Although BiPAP trials initially indicated an increased risk of myocardial infarction, more recent studies have not confirmed this concern.

When comparing CPAP and BiPAP, no significant differences were found in intubation rates or mortality. BiPAP is typically preferred for patients with chronic airway disease or acute respiratory acidosis. In practice, the choice of NIV depends on clinician familiarity with the modality.

A new approach in oxygen delivery is through high-flow nasal cannula (HFNC), which provides heated, humidified gasses at higher flow rates. While HFNC has some CPAP-like effects, studies comparing HFNC with NIV in respiratory failure have not demonstrated clear improvements in outcomes like intubation or mortality. HFNC may be considered when other NIV options are not well-tolerated.

New Pharmacological Agents

Various novel drugs have been tested for acute decompensated heart failure, including Levosimendan (a calcium sensitizer), Nesiritide (a BNP analog), and Serelaxin (a vasodilator). However, these agents have not shown consistent benefits in terms of symptom control or mortality reduction when compared to standard care, and their use may be limited by side effects such as hypotension, electrolyte imbalances, and arrhythmias. Furthermore, none of these drugs have been specifically studied for APO, so they are not recommended for use in APO patients.

Hypotensive Patients

Hypotension in APO often signals severe disease progression and cardiogenic shock, requiring both ventilatory and hemodynamic support. Intubation with rapid-sequence intubation is crucial for optimizing oxygen delivery. Positive end-expiratory pressure (PEEP) of 5–10 cm H2O may be helpful. Fluid resuscitation should be carefully titrated based on clinical response, and inotropic support with agents such as epinephrine is needed to improve cardiac output. Dobutamine can also be used, though it may lower blood pressure, requiring vasopressor use. Invasive monitoring can help guide fluid and drug therapy.

For severe cases, advanced therapeutic interventions like an intra-aortic balloon pump may be employed to reduce myocardial oxygen demand and enhance coronary perfusion. Immediate treatment of reversible causes, such as reperfusion for myocardial infarction or surgery for valvular dysfunction, is essential for improving outcomes.

Controversies

Some areas of debate in the treatment of APO include the use of natriuretic peptide levels for diagnosis, the efficacy of standard versus high-dose nitrate infusions, the optimal infusion time and dosage for diuretics like furosemide, and the potential role of new vasodilators and diuretics in treatment.

References

1. Australian Institute of Health and Welfare. Emergency Department Care 2016–17: Australian Hospital Statistics. Health Services Series No. 80. Cat. No. HSE 194. Canberra: AIHW; 2017.

2. Dawber TR, Kannel WB, Revotskie N, et al. Factors associated with the development of coronary heart disease: six-year follow-up in the Framingham study. Am J Public Health Nations Health. 1959;49(10):1349–1356.

3. Abdalla W, Elgendy M, Abdelaziz AA, Ammar MA. Lung ultrasound versus chest radiography for diagnosing pneumothorax in critically ill patients: a prospective, single-blind study. Saudi J Anaesth. 2016;10(3):265–269. https://doi.org/10.4103/1658-354X.174906.

4. Milner KA, Funk M, Richards S, et al. Symptom predictors of acute coronary syndromes in younger and older patients. Nurs Res. 2001;50(4):233–241.

5. Gräni C, Senn O, Bischof M, et al. Diagnostic performance of reproducible chest wall tenderness to rule out acute coronary syndrome in acute chest pain: a prospective diagnostic

study. BMJ Open. 2015;5(1):e007442. https://doi.org/10.1136/bmjopen-2014-007442.

6. Klompas M. Does this patient have an acute thoracic aortic dissection? JAMA. 2002;287(17):2262–2272. https://doi.org/10.1001/jama.287.17.2262.

7. Syed S, Gatien M, Perry JJ, et al. Prospective validation of a clinical decision rule to identify patients presenting with chest pain to the emergency department who can safely be removed from cardiac monitoring. CMAJ. 2017;189(4):E139–E145.

8. Thygesen K, Alpert JS, Jaffe AS, et al. Third universal definition of myocardial infarction. J Am Coll Cardiol. 2012;60(16):1581–1598. https://doi.org/10.1016/j.jacc.2012.08.001. Epub 2012 Sep 5.

9. Carlton E, Greenslade J, Cullen L, et al. Evaluation of high-sensitivity cardiac troponin I

levels in patients with suspected acute coronary syndrome. JAMA Cardiol. 2016;1(4):405–412.

10. Barraclough K, Gale CP, Hall R. Assessment of chest pain in a low-risk patient: is the exercise tolerance test obsolete? BMJ. 2015;350:h1905.

Chapter 4
Arrhythmias

Essentials

1. Urgency of Arrhythmias: Cardiac arrhythmias are critical conditions that demand prompt attention due to their potential to be life-threatening and cause sudden death.

2. Initial Evaluation: The priority in evaluating arrhythmias is assessing hemodynamic stability. For patients who are stable, a 12-lead electrocardiogram (ECG) should be conducted. In contrast, unstable patients require immediate intervention.

3. Bradyarrhythmia Evaluation: When dealing with bradyarrhythmias, it is essential to assess the patient's symptoms and correlate them with the ECG findings.

4. Wide Complex Tachycardia: Any patient presenting with wide complex tachycardia should be presumed to have ventricular tachycardia unless further investigations provide evidence to suggest otherwise.

Introduction

Arrhythmia refers to an abnormal heart rhythm, which encompasses a variety of conditions including atrial and ventricular ectopic beats. Tachycardia is characterized by a heart rate exceeding 100 beats per minute (bpm), while bradycardia is defined as a rate lower than 60 bpm. The management of arrhythmias depends on multiple factors including the patient's clinical presentation, hemodynamic stability, presence of underlying heart disease, and the specific type of arrhythmia. Stable, asymptomatic arrhythmias without underlying heart disease typically do not require emergency intervention. However, symptomatic arrhythmias, particularly those associated with structural heart disease, demand more immediate therapy. The primary objective is to restore adequate cardiac output to ensure cerebral perfusion while using interventions that minimize risk to the patient.

Pathophysiology and Pathogenesis

A clear understanding of arrhythmias requires knowledge of the heart's normal conduction system. In a healthy heart, electrical impulses originate from the sinoatrial (SA) node, propagate through the atria, and reach the atrioventricular (AV) node. From the AV node, the impulse travels down the bundle of His, then along the right and left bundle branches, and finally through the Purkinje fibers to the ventricular myocardium.

Several mechanisms can lead to arrhythmias, including re-entry, enhanced automaticity, and triggered activity. In general, arrhythmias are caused by either abnormal impulse generation or abnormal impulse conduction.

Abnormal Impulse Generation: This occurs when electrical activity arises outside the normal pacemaker cells, such as in sick sinus syndrome, where the SA node fails to initiate impulses.

Abnormal Impulse Conduction: Problems in the AV node can block the conduction of electrical signals between the atria and ventricles, resulting in varying degrees of AV block.

Ectopic Impulses: These impulses, which originate from locations other than the SA node, can cause atrial ectopics or atrial tachycardia. Additionally, accessory pathways between the atria and ventricles can lead to supraventricular tachycardia (SVT).

Ventricular Conduction Abnormalities: These include conditions like bundle branch blocks or other intraventricular conduction disturbances.

The most dangerous arrhythmias arise from the ventricles, as these can lead to sudden death, especially when underlying structural heart disease is present.

Re-entry Mechanism

Re-entry occurs when an electrical impulse circulates around a closed loop of conducting tissue, repeatedly stimulating atrial or ventricular tissue. This loop may be an anatomical abnormality, such as an accessory pathway, or a functional defect caused by ischemia or other myocardial diseases.

Enhanced and Abnormal Automaticity

Automaticity refers to the heart's ability to initiate electrical impulses without external stimulation, which is typically seen in the SA node. Enhanced automaticity occurs during conditions like exercise or drug use, which can increase impulse generation. Abnormal automaticity, however, refers to situations where impulse initiation occurs from tissue other than the SA node, such as in ventricular arrhythmias.

Triggered Activity

Triggered activity is a type of arrhythmia caused by after-depolarizations—premature depolarizations of myocardial tissue before complete repolarization. This can be early, as seen in torsades de pointes associated with a prolonged QT interval, or late, as in catecholaminergic polymorphic ventricular tachycardia and idiopathic outflow tract ventricular tachycardia.

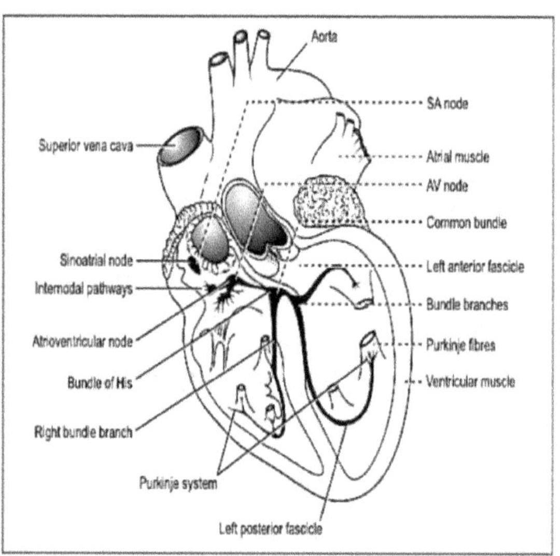

Figure 4-1: The heart's conduction system. AV represents the atrioventricular node; SA, the sinoatrial node.

Principles of Assessment and Management

Arrhythmia patients may present with symptoms such as palpitations or syncope, or may be asymptomatic, with the arrhythmia detected incidentally during routine investigations. Initial management should take place in a setting with cardiac and physiological monitoring available.

Stabilization: For all patients, initial attention should be directed towards securing the airway, breathing, and circulation.

Initial Evaluation: For stable patients, a thorough history, physical examination, and ECG are appropriate. A family history of sudden cardiac death increases suspicion of ventricular arrhythmia.

Unstable Patients: Unstable patients—those presenting with hypotension, dyspnea, chest pain, or altered consciousness—require urgent intervention to restore a stable rhythm and ensure adequate cerebral perfusion. For example, a history of renal failure or heart failure in a patient taking spironolactone may suggest that a wide complex tachycardia is secondary to hyperkalemia.

Investigations: In addition to a 12-lead ECG, blood tests (including full blood count, electrolytes, and cardiac markers) should be performed. A chest x-ray may also provide helpful diagnostic information. Depending on the clinical context, further tests such as serum digoxin levels, thyroid function tests, and theophylline levels may be necessary.

Bradyarrhythmias

Bradycardia, defined as a heart rate of fewer than 60 bpm, requires careful consideration of the patient's clinical condition. An algorithmic approach to ECG interpretation, such as the one presented in Figure 5.4.2, simplifies the diagnosis of bradyarrhythmias. In cases of denervated transplanted hearts, which do not respond to atropine, pacing and catecholamine infusion may be required.

Sinus Bradycardia

Sinus bradycardia can occur due to physiological factors (such as in athletes), drug effects (e.g., β-blockers or calcium channel blockers), or vagal stimulation (e.g., during vomiting). More concerning causes include acute inferior myocardial infarction, raised intracranial pressure, hypothermia, and hypothyroidism.

Clinical Features: Symptoms are often absent but may arise depending on the underlying cause.

ECG Features: The atrial rate equals the ventricular rate, with a normal PR interval and P-wave morphology.

Management: Treatment focuses on addressing the underlying cause. If there are signs of hypoperfusion, intravenous atropine (0.5 mg) can be administered while the cause is being investigated. Physiological bradycardia generally does not require treatment, and management depends on the underlying condition.

Sick Sinus Syndrome (Bradycardia-Tachycardia Syndrome)

Sick sinus syndrome is most commonly seen in elderly patients and results from fibrosis around the sinus node. It can also arise from congenital heart disease, rheumatic disorders, myocarditis, pericarditis, cardiomyopathies, and ischemic heart disease. This syndrome is marked by sinus bradycardia with intermittent sinus node dysfunction, leading to periods of prolonged pauses followed by escape rhythms. Conditions like thyrotoxicosis, hyperkalemia, and certain medications (e.g., β-blockers, digoxin) can exacerbate the syndrome.

Clinical Features

Patients may present with symptoms such as fainting (syncope), dizziness, palpitations, shortness of breath, chest discomfort, collapse, or cerebrovascular events.

Clinical Investigations and ECG Findings

ECG Characteristics

Sinus bradycardia: Abnormally slow heart rate due to reduced sinus node activity.

Intermittent absence of P waves: Periods where atrial depolarization fails, leading to pauses.

Long pauses with escape rhythms: Prolonged gaps followed by slower back-up heart rhythms.

Return of sinus activity: A natural resumption of normal heart pacing after pauses.

Treatment

For unstable patients:

1. Administer intravenous atropine (0.5 mg IV) to temporarily increase heart rate until pacing.

2. If ineffective, consider adrenaline (2–10 μg/min) or dopamine (2–10 μg/kg/min) infusions if pacing is delayed.

3. Use transcutaneous pacing if medications fail.

Avoid medications for rapid heart rhythms (tachyarrhythmias) in cases of pre-existing heart block until pacemaker insertion, as they can exacerbate the condition. Ultimately, patients will need a permanent pacemaker.

Heart Block Types and Their Management

1. First-Degree Atrioventricular (AV) Block

Characterized by a delayed transmission of impulses from the atria to the ventricles, leading to a prolonged PR interval (>0.2 seconds). Causes may include:

Medications, vagal stimulation, myocardial infarction, or high vagal tone in young, healthy individuals.

ECG Features

P wave consistently followed by QRS: Each atrial contraction leads to ventricular contraction.

PR interval >200 ms: Constant and prolonged PR interval.

Asymptomatic patients do not require specific treatment or hospitalization.

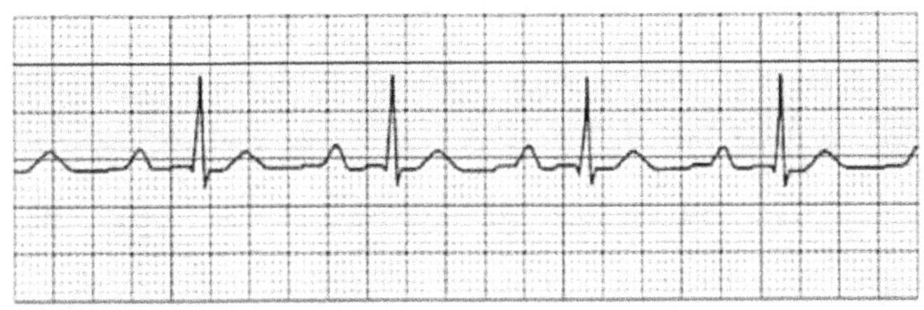

Figure 4-2: Rhythm strip showing first-degree atrioventricular block.

Figure 4-3: Rhythm strip illustrating second-degree atrioventricular block, Mobitz type.

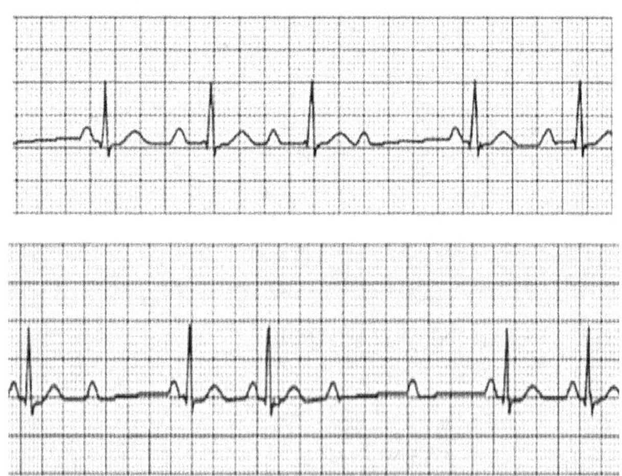

Figure 4.4: Rhythm strip showing second-degree atrioventricular block, Mobitz II type.

2. Second-Degree AV Block

Mobitz Type I (Wenckebach)

Here, progressive elongation of the PR interval occurs until a QRS complex is dropped. Causes include myocardial infarction, medications, or high vagal tone.

ECG Features

Gradual PR interval lengthening until dropped QRS.

Grouped beating.

Treatment

Typically, no treatment is needed if stable. For instability, administer atropine, dopamine/adrenaline infusion, or consider pacing.

Mobitz Type II

This type is characterized by constant PR intervals with intermittent failure of P waves conducting to QRS. The block is typically below the AV node, often in the bundle of His or branches, and may cause symptoms.

ECG Features

Atrial rate > ventricular rate.

Regular atrial rhythm with dropped QRS complexes.

Immediate intervention includes IV atropine if unstable. Consider adrenaline or dopamine if pacing is delayed. Hospital admission is required as this can progress to complete heart block.

3. Third-Degree (Complete) AV Block

In complete AV block, there is a total dissociation between atrial and ventricular activity. Backup pacemakers activate either within or below the AV node, resulting in narrow or wide QRS complexes, respectively.

ECG Features

Complete AV dissociation.

Escape pacemaker rate between 20-50 bpm.

For hemodynamically unstable patients, administer atropine 0.5 mg IV and consider dopamine or adrenaline infusions. External pacing may be necessary. Admission and eventual permanent pacing are required.

Warning: Avoid medications like lignocaine that could suppress ventricular escape rhythms in complete AV block, as this could decrease cardiac output.

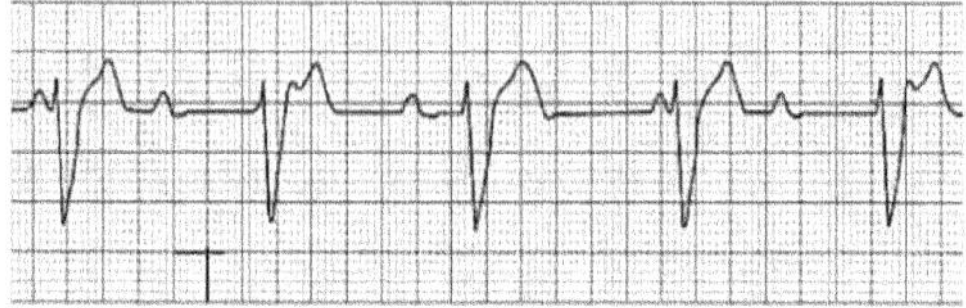

Figure 4-5: Rhythm strip showing a narrow complex third-degree heart block.

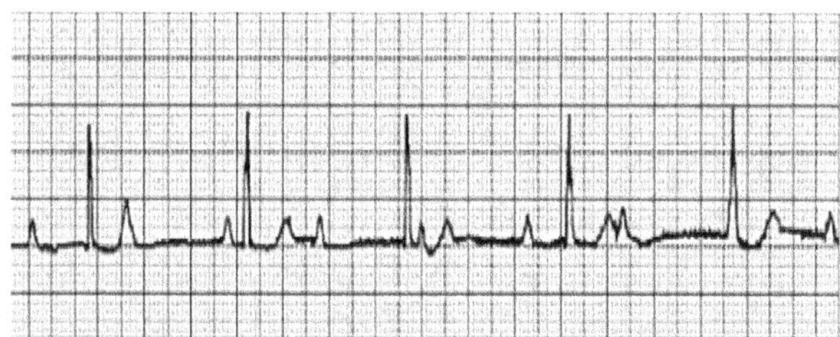

Figure 4-6: Rhythm strip illustrating third-degree heart block.

Tachyarrhythmias: Diagnostic Approach

Diagnosing tachyarrhythmias often relies on evaluating QRS width and rhythm regularity. Broad complex tachycardia, often treated as ventricular tachycardia (VT) unless proven otherwise, is common in older patients with ischemic heart disease and symptoms like syncope.

Management of Ventricular Tachycardias (VT)

VT requires correct identification and immediate management, especially in unstable patients. Treatment involves synchronized cardioversion and addressing any underlying electrolyte imbalances. Stable VT patients should undergo a 12-lead ECG for detailed rhythm analysis.

Monomorphic Ventricular Tachycardia (VT)

Sustained VT is identified as a sequence of ventricular impulses exceeding 100 bpm, lasting over 30 seconds, or leading to hemodynamic instability. For hemodynamically stable patients, a 12-lead ECG should be obtained to analyze the rhythm's morphology.

Symptoms:

Patients may have palpitations, dizziness, chest discomfort, or may be asymptomatic. Notable signs include cannon 'a' waves in neck veins and potential loss of consciousness.

ECG Characteristics (Refer to Figure 4-7 and 4-8):

AV Dissociation

Fusion or Capture Beats

QRS Complex Width: >140 ms

Heart Rate: Typically 150–200 bpm, consistently above 100 bpm

Regular Rhythm with occasional variability

QRS Axis: Often left or northwest axis deviation

RBBB Morphology VT: Deep S wave, r/S ratio <1

AV dissociation and fusion or capture beats, though uncommon at faster rates, are definitive for VT if observed.

Treatment Protocol

VT management follows AHA/ACC guidelines. Pulseless VT protocols are covered in Section 1. For all VT patients, administer oxygen and establish IV access while collecting blood for electrolyte and cardiac marker analysis. Correct any electrolyte abnormalities, particularly potassium.

Unstable Patients: Immediate cardioversion, with sedation if needed. Start with 100 J synchronized DC shock, escalating as necessary (150 J, 200 J, 360 J). For biphasic defibrillators, use equivalent energy levels (e.g., 70 J, 120 J, 150 J, 170 J). If VT persists after shocks, initiate amiodarone as the primary treatment, with lignocaine, magnesium, or procainamide as secondary options. An infusion of amiodarone or lignocaine should follow cardioversion. If blood pressure remains low, consider inotropic support (e.g., dopamine). For cases where cardiac causes are suspected, consider urgent coronary angiography, regardless of the absence of ST elevation or chest pain.

Stable Patients: Administer IV amiodarone, 150 mg slowly over 10 minutes, with a second dose if needed. Alternatively, IV procainamide can be given (100 mg every 5 minutes, up to 10–20 mg/kg).

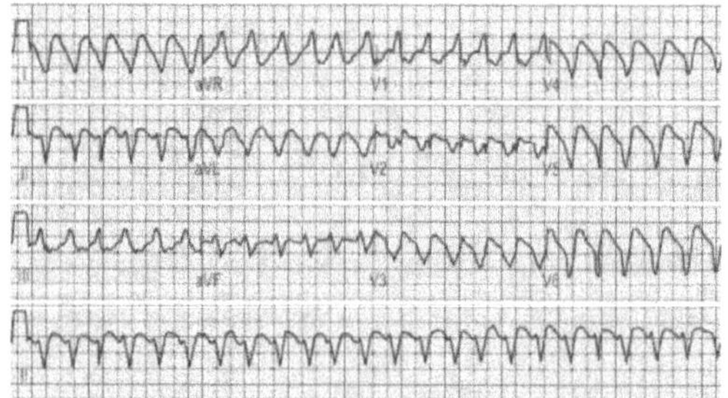

Figure 4-7: Ventricular tachycardia.

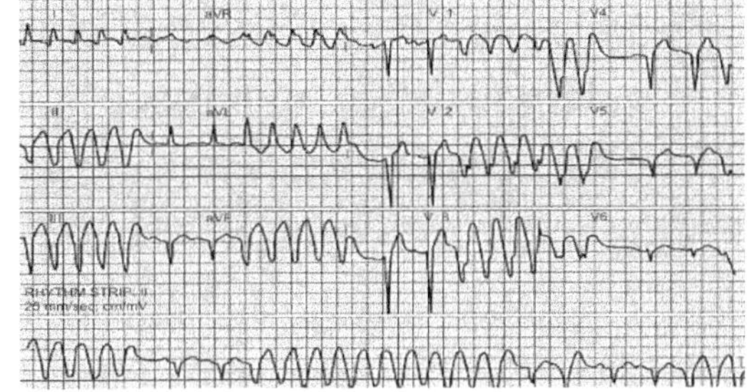

Figure. 4-8: Non-sustained ventricular tachycardia.

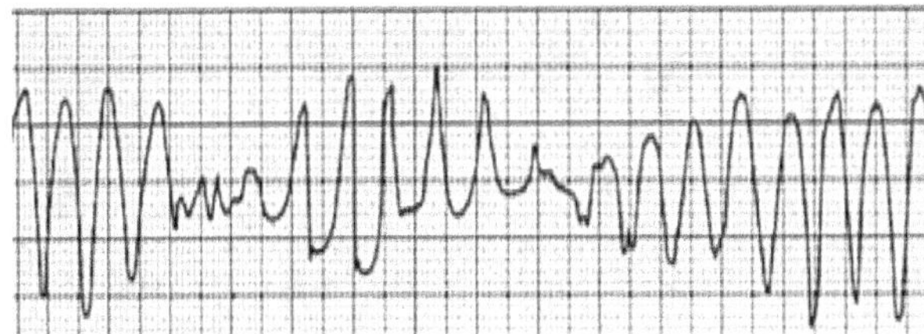

Figure 4-9 Torsades de pointes.

Management and Characteristics of Different Ventricular Tachycardias (VT) and Related Tachyarrhythmias

Monomorphic Ventricular Tachycardia (VT)

Sustained monomorphic VT is defined as a series of rapid ventricular impulses occurring at over 100 beats per minute, persisting for more than 30 seconds, or causing hemodynamic instability. In stable cases, a 12-lead ECG is recommended to define the morphology. Patients may experience palpitations, dizziness, or chest pain and may exhibit cannon "a" waves in the neck veins or lose consciousness.

ECG Features:

AV dissociation, fusion beats, or capture beats

Wide QRS complexes (>140 ms)

Heart rate typically between 150-200 bpm

Regular rhythm with minor beat-to-beat variation

Consistent QRS axis, frequently with left or northwest axis deviation

Deep S waves in RBBB morphology with r/S ratio <1

Treatment: All patients with VT should receive oxygen, IV access, and an electrolyte assessment. In unstable patients, immediate synchronized cardioversion with escalating energy is needed. Amiodarone is recommended for VT resistant to shock, while adjunctive options like lignocaine, magnesium, and procainamide may also be used.

Polymorphic Ventricular Tachycardia (Polymorphic VT)

Characterized by a QRS complex with continuously changing morphology, polymorphic VT is often associated with ischemia and is generally more electrically unstable than monomorphic VT. Torsades de Pointes, a subtype linked to prolonged QT, shows a twisting QRS pattern.

ECG Features:

Rapid, wide QRS complexes with varying morphology

Irregular rhythm in some cases

Treatment: Administer magnesium sulfate for torsades de pointes and consider overdrive pacing. Cardioversion is advised if the patient is unstable, with correction of the underlying cause being crucial.

Idiopathic Ventricular Tachycardia (VT)

Idiopathic VT is monomorphic and occurs without structural heart disease. The QRS morphology during tachycardia helps localize its origin.

Types and ECG Characteristics:

Right Ventricular Outflow Tract (RVOT) VT: Left bundle branch block (LBBB) with inferior axis.

Idiopathic Left Ventricular Tachycardia (ILVT): RBBB pattern with left axis deviation and QRS duration between 100-140 ms.

Propranolol-Sensitive Monomorphic VT: May present with either LBBB or RBBB morphology.

Management: Response to beta-blockers, verapamil, and adenosine is typical for RVOT VT. Catheter ablation is highly effective for ILVT, especially when vagal maneuvers and adenine are ineffective.

Pre-Excited Atrial Fibrillation (WPW Syndrome)

Pre-excited AF, often linked with Wolff-Parkinson-White (WPW) syndrome, is characterized by an irregular, wide complex tachycardia in patients younger than 50 years, often with a history of palpitations.

ECG Features:

Rapid ventricular rate (>180 bpm), bypassing normal AV node conduction

Wide, abnormal QRS complexes indicative of aberrant conduction

Narrow QRS complexes occasionally seen when conducting through the AV node

Treatment: Immediate cardioversion is indicated for hemodynamically unstable patients. In stable patients, procainamide or ibutilide can be used. Certain agents, like adenosine, amiodarone, and verapamil, should be avoided due to the risk of precipitating ventricular fibrillation.

Supraventricular Tachycardia (SVT) with Aberrant Conduction

In patients with pre-existing bundle branch block (BBB), SVT may appear as a wide-complex tachycardia. Unlike WPW, SVT with aberrant conduction shows a stable QRS morphology beat-to-beat.

Narrow Complex Tachycardias

Sinus tachycardia, with a rate exceeding 100 bpm, may be caused by various factors like shock, hypoxia, heart failure, or fever. Symptoms may include palpitations, but clinical signs are generally associated with the underlying cause.

ECG Features:

Regular rhythm with a rate of 100-160 bpm

Uniform P waves preceding each QRS complex

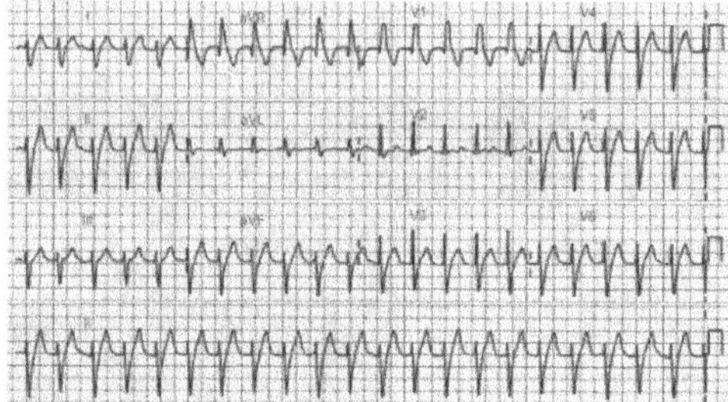

Figure 4-10: Idiopathic left ventricular tachycardia.

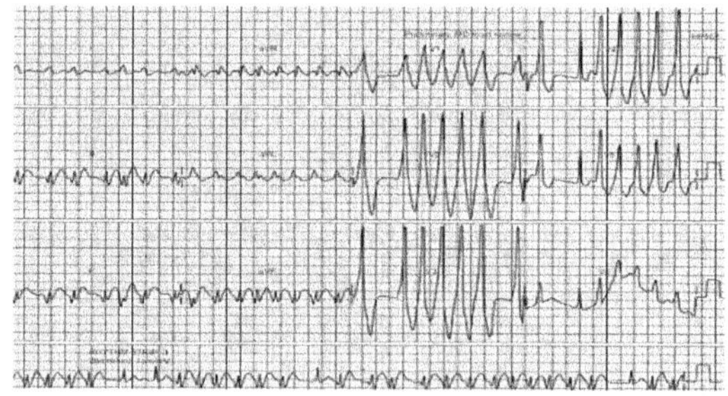

Figure 4-11: Pre-excited atrial fibrillation

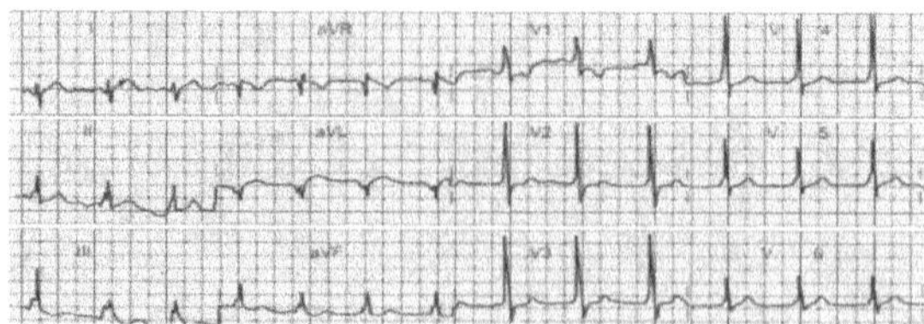

Figure 4-12: Wolff-Parkinson-White syndrome: 12-lead electrocardiogram showing δ waves

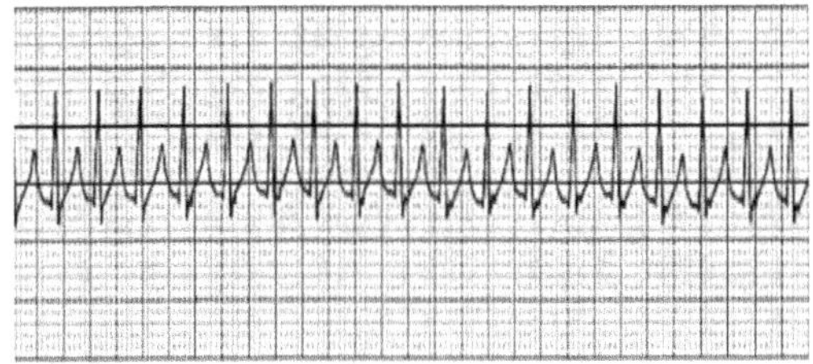

Figure 4-13: Paroxysmal supraventricular tachycardia.

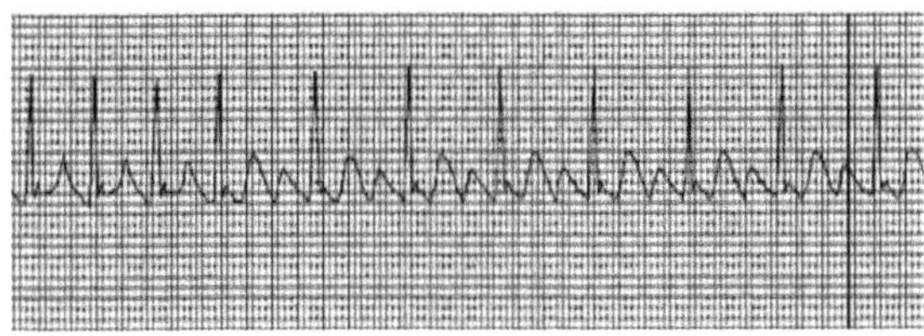

Figure 4-14: Rhythm strip of atrial flutter.

Wolff-Parkinson-White (WPW) Syndrome

WPW syndrome, the most prevalent of the accessory pathway syndromes, results from an additional conductive muscle bridge known as the bundle of Kent. This pathway connects the atria and ventricles, bypassing the AV node. When in sinus rhythm, the ECG often shows a PR interval under 0.12 seconds, a delta wave (characterized by a slurred upstroke), and a wide QRS complex exceeding 0.10 seconds.

Clinical Presentation

Patients may report symptoms like palpitations, chest pain, or syncope.

ECG Characteristics

Rate: 150 to 250 bpm

Rhythm: Regular

P Waves: Atrial P waves appear distinct from sinus P waves. These are typically visible at lower rates but become indistinct at higher rates (over 200 bpm), sometimes merging with the preceding T wave.

PR Interval: Often unmeasurable due to the P wave blending with the T wave. If measurable, it typically ranges from 0.12 to 0.20 seconds.

QRS Duration: Less than 0.10 seconds

For acute treatment of regular paroxysmal supraventricular tachycardia (PSVT), vagal maneuvers and intravenous adenosine are first-line therapies. For hemodynamically unstable patients, cardioversion is necessary, generally with sedation. For those stable yet unresponsive to initial treatments, options include intravenous beta-blockers, diltiazem, or verapamil. Flecainide may serve as third-line therapy. Resistant cases may require electrical cardioversion.

Atrial Flutter

Risk factors mirror those of atrial fibrillation (AF), including thyrotoxicosis, obesity, obstructive sleep apnea, pulmonary disease, and others. Symptoms may include palpitations or chest pain, although many patients remain asymptomatic.

ECG Features

Rate: Atrial rate typically 250-350 bpm, often around 300 bpm. The ventricular rate is variable, usually around 150 bpm with a 2:1 AV block, though other block patterns may occur.

Rhythm: Regular atrial rhythm, with the ventricular rhythm often regular but sometimes irregular.

P Waves: Characteristic "sawtooth" flutter waves, best observed in leads II, III, and aVF.

PR Interval: Not measurable

QRS Duration: Typically under 0.10 seconds but may be widened if flutter waves overlap with the QRS complex

Hemodynamically unstable patients respond to low-energy cardioversion or intravenous amiodarone. Stable patients may benefit from synchronized cardioversion, rapid atrial pacing, or medications like IV beta-blockers, diltiazem, or verapamil for rate control.

Atrial Fibrillation (AF)

AF arises from chaotic atrial depolarization due to multiple re-entry pathways, leading to an uncoordinated atrial activity. AF has an irregular rhythm with absent discrete P waves and may be either acute or chronic. Common ED causes include electrolyte imbalances and hyperthyroidism, as listed in medical guidelines.

Types of AF

1. Paroxysmal AF

2. AF with slow ventricular response

3. AF with rapid ventricular response

Clinical Symptoms

Acute AF episodes may cause palpitations, dyspnea, dizziness, or angina. Chronic AF is often asymptomatic, particularly when the heart rate is under 100 bpm. The clinical hallmark is an irregularly irregular pulse.

ECG Features

P Waves: Absent

Baseline: Chaotic, irregular with fibrillatory waves

RR Cycles: Irregularly irregular

QRS Duration: Intermittently widened due to aberrant conduction

Management

The treatment approach varies by the AF duration, hemodynamic stability, ventricular rate, and underlying structural heart disease. Urgent electrical cardioversion is recommended for unstable patients with rapid ventricular response. For those hemodynamically stable, options include immediate or delayed cardioversion and rate control. Anticoagulation decisions are based on the CHADS-VASc score. A rhythm-control strategy may suit younger patients without structural disease, while rate control is generally preferred for older patients and those with contraindications. Pharmacologic cardioversion may involve amiodarone, flecainide, or other antiarrhythmics, while rate control can be achieved with beta-blockers, verapamil, or diltiazem.

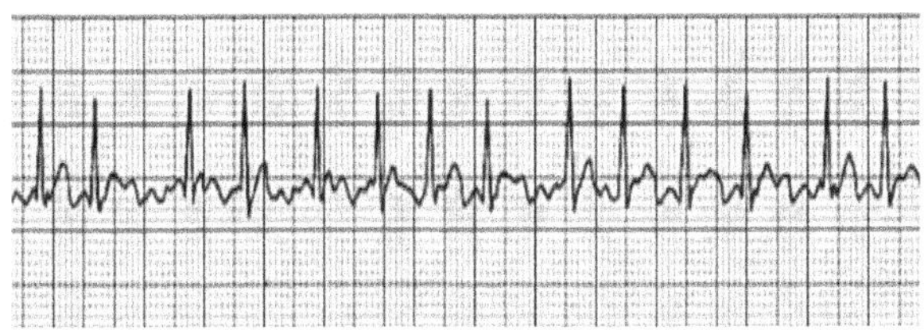

Figure 4-15: Rhythm strip of atrial fibrillation.

Multifocal Atrial Tachycardia (MAT)

MAT is an arrhythmia marked by at least three different P-wave morphologies, a heart rate over

100 bpm, and variable PP, PR, and RR intervals. Commonly linked to chronic obstructive pulmonary disease and electrolyte imbalances, its treatment focuses on managing the underlying condition, with IV magnesium providing some benefit.

Trifascicular Blocks

A bifascicular block impedes one infranodal pathway, such as the right bundle branch block (RBBB), left anterior fascicular block (LAFB), or left posterior fascicular block (LPFB).

ECG Patterns

LAFB: Left-axis deviation with a normal QRS duration

LPFB: Right-axis deviation with a normal QRS duration

RBBB: Often a normal variant, with an rSR pattern in V1 and V2, broad S waves in left leads, and a QRS >120 ms in complete blocks

Management targets the underlying cause, with additional workup required for new-onset RBBB.

Left Bundle Branch Block (LBBB)
Typically pathological, LBBB is associated with coronary artery disease, ischemia, hypertension, myocarditis, and cardiomyopathies.

ECG Findings

R Waves: Broad, notched, or slurred in leads I, aVL, V5, and V6

QRS Duration: >120 ms

The Sgarbossa criteria may help detect ST-elevation myocardial infarction (STEMI) in LBBB patients, with key indicators including concordant ST elevation, ST depression in V1-V3, and discordant ST elevation.

Combination Blocks

A bifascicular block involves blockage of two infranodal pathways. Specific diagnostic and treatment strategies vary based on the pathways involved and patient presentation.

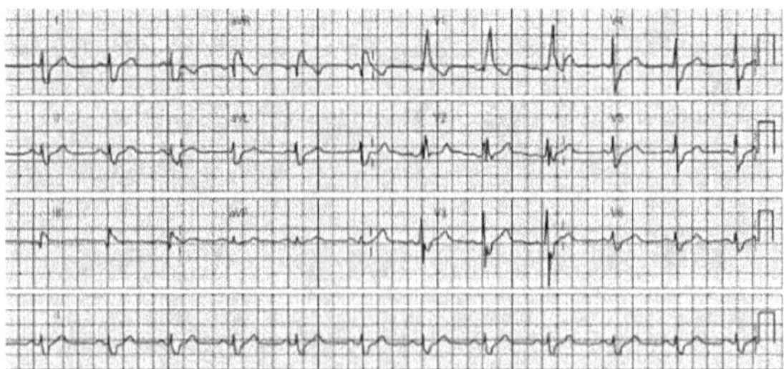

Figure 4-16 Right bundle branch block

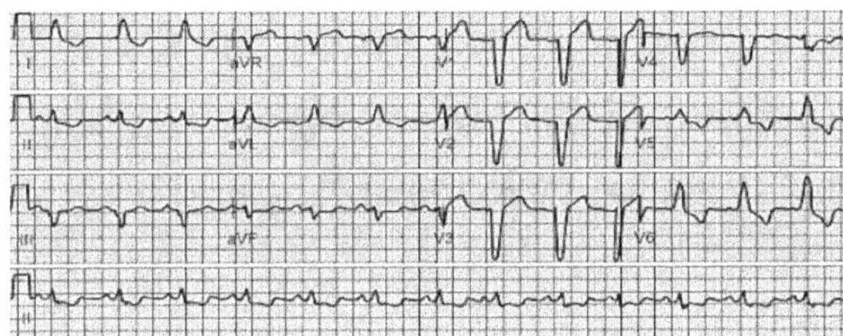

Figure 4-17: Left bundle branch block

The QRS complex is typically normal unless it is aberrantly conducted. If it occurs early, it may be blocked, indicating a blocked atrial ectopic, but in most cases, treatment is not required.

Junctional Rhythm

Junctional rhythm is generally asymptomatic. The ECG characteristics of this rhythm are as follows:

The rate is slower than the sinus rhythm.

The rhythm is regular.

There is no preceding P wave.

Occasionally, the P wave may appear before or immediately after the QRS complex (with inverted P waves in leads II, III, and aVF).

The QRS complex is usually narrow unless it is aberrantly conducted.
In most cases, no treatment is necessary.

Brugada Syndrome

Brugada syndrome is characterized by right bundle branch block morphology on the ECG, accompanied by ST-segment elevation in leads V1 and V2, along with terminal T wave inversion. Symptoms may include syncope or cardiac arrest. It is crucial to distinguish the Brugada pattern from Brugada syndrome, as the ECG pattern with accompanying symptoms may be linked to sudden cardiac death due to ventricular fibrillation, often with a family history of sudden death. Brugada syndrome is a channelopathy, and in some instances, the ECG pattern may appear only during fever or following the use of antiarrhythmic drugs, particularly class IC agents like flecainide or propafenone. Patients displaying the Brugada pattern should be referred for further evaluation and risk stratification.

Controversies

There is limited evidence from randomized controlled trials regarding the effectiveness of many second-line antiarrhythmic drugs.

The role of observation for minimally symptomatic recent-onset paroxysmal arrhythmias is still debated.

References

1. Callaway CW, Soar J, Aibiki M, et al. Advanced Life Support Chapter Collaborators. Part 4: Advanced life support: 2015 international consensus on cardiopulmonary resuscitation and emergency cardiovascular care science with

treatment recommendations. Circulation. 2015;132(suppl 1):S84–S145.

2. Page RL, Joglar JA, Caldwell MA, et al. 2015 ACC/AHA/HRS guideline for the management of adult patients with supraventricular tachycardia: A report of the American College of Cardiology/American Heart Association Task Force on Clinical Practice Guidelines and the Heart Rhythm Society. J Am Coll Cardiol. 2016;67:e27–e115.

3. January CT, Wann LS, Alpert JS, et al. 2014 AHA/ACC/HRS guideline for the management of patients with atrial fibrillation: A report of the American College of Cardiology/American Heart Association Task Force on Practice Guidelines and the Heart Rhythm Society. Circulation. 2014;130(23):e199–e267.

4. Atzema CL, Barrett TW. Managing atrial fibrillation. Ann Emerg Med. 2015;65:532–539.

5. Sgarbossa EB, Pinski SL, Barbagelata A, et al. Electrocardiographic diagnosis of evolving acute myocardial infarction in the presence of left bundle-branch block. GUSTO-1 (Global Utilization of Streptokinase and Tissue Plasminogen Activator for Occluded Coronary Arteries) Investigators. N Eng J Med. 1996;334:481–487.

6. Sgarbossa EB, Pinski SL, Wagner GS. Left bundle-branch block and the ECG in diagnosis of acute myocardial infarction. J Am Med Assoc. 1999;282:1224–1225.

7. Shah CP, Thakur RK, Xie B, et al. Clinical approach to wide complex tachycardias. Emerg Clin North Am. 1998;16:331–359.

8. Stiell IG, Macle L. CCS atrial fibrillation guidelines committee. Canadian Cardiovascular Society atrial fibrillation guidelines 2010: Management of recent onset atrial fibrillation and flutter in the emergency department. Can J Cardiol. 2011;27:38–46.

9. Shen W-K, Sheldon RS, Benditt DG, et al. 2017 ACC/AHA/HRS guideline for the evaluation and management of patients with syncope: A report of the American College of Cardiology/American Heart Association Task Force on Clinical Practice Guidelines and the Heart Rhythm Society. J Am Coll Cardiol. 2017;70:e39–e110.

10. Al-Khatib SM, Stevenson WG, Ackerman MJ, et al. 2017 AHA/ACC/HRS guideline for management of patients with ventricular arrhythmias and the prevention of sudden cardiac death: A report of the American College of Cardiology Foundation/American Heart Association Task Force on Clinical Practice Guidelines and the Heart Rhythm Society. Circulation. 2018;138(13):e272–e391.

Chapter 5
Pulmonary embolism

Essentials

1. Venous thromboembolism (VTE) encompasses a range of clinical presentations, progressing from deep venous thrombosis (DVT) to the more severe and potentially fatal complication of pulmonary embolism (PE).

2. If left untreated, PE carries a high risk of recurrence and mortality, but this risk is significantly reduced with appropriate anticoagulation therapy.

3. Diagnostic and treatment strategies should be guided by effective risk assessment, ideally using validated tools such as the Wells criteria and the Pulmonary Embolism Rule-Out Criteria (PERC), to minimize unnecessary tests and treatments while effectively managing patients.

4. The diagnostic approach should include electrocardiography (ECG), chest X-ray (CXR), oxygenation assessments, and additional tests to rule out alternative diagnoses. Computed tomography pulmonary angiography (CTPA) remains the primary diagnostic tool. Other tests, including age-adjusted D-dimer, lower limb ultrasound, ventilation/perfusion (V/Q) scan, and single-photon emission computed tomography (SPECT), may be used to refine diagnosis, depending on available resources.

5. Treatment decisions are based on a diagnostic threshold (over 80% likelihood of PE), where the benefits of anticoagulation outweigh the associated risks.

6. For massive (hemodynamically unstable) PE, the initial diagnostic approach should include transthoracic echocardiography or, when available, trans-esophageal echocardiography.

7. Direct oral anticoagulants (DOACs) are the first-line treatment for most PE cases, although some sub-segmental PE (SSPE) cases may not require treatment.

8. Thrombolysis (or embolectomy, if thrombolysis is contraindicated or ineffective) is reserved for hemodynamically unstable patients. Stable patients with signs of right ventricular strain should be closely monitored, with urgent thrombolysis initiated if they clinically deteriorate.

9. Prognosis should be evaluated using combined clinical and diagnostic factors, with tools like the Simplified Pulmonary Embolism Severity Index (SPESI) to inform management and patient disposition.

Introduction

Pulmonary embolism (PE) is a prevalent cardiovascular condition, ranking third in frequency, particularly affecting the elderly with coexisting comorbidities such as cancer, trauma, immobility, recent surgery, or severe medical conditions. Historically, untreated PE has a high mortality rate, but anticoagulation therapy has significantly reduced in-hospital mortality to between 4% and 12%.

Diagnosing and managing PE presents numerous challenges, as it requires thorough clinical evaluation, validated risk assessment (e.g., Wells or PERC scores), and careful selection of diagnostic tests, none of which are definitive. It is essential to consider alternative conditions with similar symptoms. Diagnostic tests for PE, including D-dimer, should be used cautiously and based on risk assessment to avoid unnecessary testing and minimize false positives. In patients with low PE risk (<5%), an alternative diagnosis should be prioritized unless no other condition is identified, while overzealous radiological testing in low-risk patients can result in false positives for venous thromboembolism (VTE). In contrast, a PE probability of 70% to 80% warrants treatment due to the clear benefit outweighing the risks. Diagnostic guidelines typically employ the Wells and/or PERC scores, with D-dimer used for low-risk patients, followed by imaging (CT pulmonary angiography [CTPA] or occasionally nuclear ventilation/perfusion scan [V/Q]). Further testing, such as venous ultrasound or CT venography, may be needed if the results are inconclusive. Echocardiography, when available, aids in risk stratification and managing unstable patients.

Anticoagulation is almost always initiated in PE cases, with most patients receiving direct oral anticoagulants (DOACs) or novel oral anticoagulants (NOACs), while others may receive heparin or warfarin. In cases of massive PE with shock (e.g., BP <90 mm Hg for over 15 minutes or requiring inotropic support), thrombolysis or embolectomy is recommended. Submassive PE generally does not warrant thrombolysis. Disposition decisions, such as whether to continue treatment at home or under intensive monitoring, are guided by prognostic tools like the Simplified Pulmonary Embolism Severity Index (SPESI), PE severity markers (e.g., brain natriuretic peptide [BNP], troponin), or echocardiography.

Aetiology, Pathogenesis, and Pathology

Approximately 30% of PE cases, particularly those seen in emergency departments, are idiopathic. Risk factors typically involve more than one component of Virchow's triad (vessel wall injury, venous stasis, and hypercoagulability). The main risk factors for secondary (provoked) PE include:

Surgery or trauma (particularly pelvic/lower abdominal, lower limb, or central nervous system surgery, which accounts for 15% to 30% of PE cases)

Cancer (15% to 25%)

Systemic diseases with immobilization, especially heart disease and strokes (15% to 25%)

A history of deep venous thrombosis (DVT)/PE, particularly unprovoked cases (5% to 15%)

PE incidence increases significantly with age, with individuals over 85 years old exhibiting a rate much higher than those between 18 and 25, largely due to comorbidities. Hypercoagulable states, such as deficiencies in antithrombin III, factor V Leiden, and protein C/S, as well as conditions like antiphospholipid syndrome, obesity, hormone therapy, and certain autoimmune diseases, elevate the risk of PE. Other factors include smoking, use of nonsteroidal anti-inflammatory drugs (NSAIDs), and prolonged immobility, such as during long-haul flights.

Prevention

Surgical procedures are the leading preventable cause of DVT and PE. Other common causes of venous stasis, such as prolonged bed rest due to illness (especially in cancer, stroke, or cardiopulmonary diseases), also contribute significantly to the development of PE. Preventative measures, including the administration of low-dose low-molecular-weight heparin (LMWH) or NOACs/DOACs, help reduce the risk of PE and improve outcomes for high-risk hospitalized medical patients. Thromboprophylaxis risk assessments should be conducted as early as possible.

Clinical Features

History

A thorough history is crucial for diagnosing PE. Most patients present with sudden-onset dyspnea, often recurring or rapid, or chest pain of any type. Syncope, especially when accompanied by respiratory symptoms or signs, suggests severe disease. Deep vein thrombosis (DVT) symptoms should be sought in all PE patients. Hemoptysis, although uncommon, may offer some predictive value. Identifying associated risk factors—divided into major and minor categories—helps increase the likelihood of PE and should be incorporated into the risk assessment process.

Examination

Physical signs supporting a PE diagnosis are rare, though certain findings can significantly increase the likelihood of PE. These include persistent unexplained tachycardia (>100 beats per minute at rest), which is commonly incorporated into prediction rules. Signs of DVT, such as a swollen leg with pain or thrombophlebitis, elevate PE risk and require imaging. Other signs, such as tachypnea (50% to 80%), cough (10% to 20%), mild fever (<38.5°C), and pleural effusion/rub, are not specific to PE. Occasionally, elevated jugular venous pressure (JVP) or abnormal heart sounds suggest right ventricular strain, which can indicate PE.

Risk Assessment for the Diagnosis of Pulmonary Embolism

Pre-test probability (PTP) assessment, based on history, clinical examination, and initial investigations (e.g., chest X-ray, arterial blood gasses, ECG), is essential in guiding the diagnostic strategy. For non-experts, validated scoring systems are the most effective method for estimating PTP. The Wells score is the most widely used and validated tool for assessing PE risk. If the Wells score is low (<2), the PERC score is used to determine whether D-dimer testing is necessary. If PERC is negative, PE can be excluded (<2% incidence) without further testing. If PERC is positive in low-risk patients, age-adjusted D-dimer levels are evaluated, followed by imaging if indicated. For higher-risk patients (Wells >4), D-dimer testing is bypassed, and imaging is performed directly.

Anticoagulation Before Diagnosis

In high-risk PE patients (Wells >6), anticoagulation should be initiated with direct oral anticoagulants (DOACs), LMWH, unfractionated heparin (UFH), or fondaparinux, unless contraindications exist. For intermediate-risk patients, the decision to begin anticoagulation before diagnosis should weigh the potential benefits against the bleeding risks, especially in the presence of severe underlying conditions. All unstable patients, including those with hypoxia, tachycardia, hypotension, or elevated lactate levels, should receive immediate anticoagulation unless absolute contraindications exist, alongside thrombolysis or embolectomy as necessary.

Imaging

A normal chest X-ray with significant hypoxia can be suggestive of PE, although the X-ray is abnormal in 80% to 90% of cases. In cases of confirmed PE, signs such as an enlarged pulmonary artery, pulmonary oligemia, or a Hampton hump (a characteristic semi-circular opacity) are highly specific. However, these findings may be subtle and often require retrospective identification. The primary role of the chest X-ray is to rule out other conditions and guide the decision to perform a V/Q scan.

Electrocardiography

Electrocardiogram (ECG) findings for PE are varied and generally lack sensitivity and specificity. The most significant ECG abnormalities associated with PE include tachycardia (especially atrial), right bundle branch block, right axis deviation, T-wave inversions (particularly in leads V1-V3), and the S1Q3T3 pattern, although these are not definitive indicators of PE.

Pulmonary Embolism Diagnosis and Management

Imaging Considerations in Pulmonary Embolism (PE) Diagnosis:

When assessing patients for pulmonary embolism (PE), it is important to consider various imaging modalities, with each offering distinct advantages and limitations based on clinical factors.

1. CT Pulmonary Angiography (CTPA)

CTPA is widely used in the diagnosis of PE, offering high diagnostic accuracy. However, in men with proliferative breast tissue, radiation doses (2 to 4 Gy per breast) may significantly elevate lifetime breast cancer risks (1 in 1000 per CTPA). For female patients, particularly perimenopausal or pregnant women, V/Q scanning and/or ultrasound (US) of the legs should be the preferred diagnostic method to minimize fetal radiation exposure. Both CTPA and V/Q scans present minimal fetal radiation risk if proper precautions are followed.

2. Ventilation/Perfusion (V/Q) Scanning

V/Q scanning, available in most tertiary centers, is beneficial for patients with renal dysfunction or dye allergies. While complications are rare, V/Q scanning involves moderate radiation exposure. A major limitation is the extended time required for patients to undergo the scan in often distant nuclear medicine departments, as most centers do not offer 24/7 scanning. Additionally, more than 50% of V/Q scans in the PIOPED study were non-diagnostic without proper risk assessment. Patients with visible chest X-ray (CXR) abnormalities or major lung diseases may also present with indeterminate V/Q scans and should instead undergo CTPA.

Two pivotal studies—PIOPED and McMaster—have classified V/Q scan results into four categories: normal, low, intermediate, or high probability, based on the number and size of unperfused lung segments. These results guide management decisions, as outlined below:

Normal/Near-Normal Scan: Excludes significant PE, with a 14% occurrence in the PIOPED study.

High-Probability Scan: Suggests PE in over 85% of cases but carries a 15% false-positive rate. For patients with low pretest risk, further testing is advised.

Low and Intermediate-Probability: Found in 42% and 36% of PIOPED patients, respectively. PE likelihood varies, with low-risk patients often safely discharged after excluding other major diagnoses. Further imaging may be necessary for those with critical cardiorespiratory issues due to the high mortality risk associated with even a small PE.

Low vs. High-Risk or Intermediate vs. Intermediate Results: These patients may require further imaging with CTPA and/or leg imaging to confirm or exclude PE.

3. V/Q SPECT (Single Photon Emission Computed Tomography)

V/Q SPECT combines V/Q scanning with low-dose CT for three-dimensional lung imaging, improving image clarity and allowing better delineation of perfusion defects. This method has been shown to be more accurate than traditional planar V/Q scanning, with diagnostic accuracy ranging from 90% to 98%. V/Q SPECT provides definitive PE diagnosis or exclusion and is considered an acceptable alternative when CTPA results are inconclusive. Additionally, its combination with CT offers improved specificity by identifying lung abnormalities that may cause perfusion defects. Although limited studies have directly compared V/Q SPECT to CTPA, it is becoming increasingly available in nuclear medicine departments.

4. Magnetic Resonance Imaging (MRI)

MRI is rarely indicated in PE diagnosis due to its limited role in this context.

5. Echocardiography (Transthoracic or Transoesophageal)

Echocardiography is useful for diagnosing massive PE in unstable patients by excluding other causes of hypotension, such as cardiac tamponade or myocardial dysfunction. It can demonstrate signs of right heart distension and dysfunction, which are indicative of a massive PE. Echocardiography is also important for guiding thrombolytic therapy decisions in unstable patients. However, it is less sensitive for diagnosing non-massive PE or peripheral emboli, and therefore not recommended for stable patients. The presence of right ventricular strain on echocardiography correlates with a higher risk of poor outcomes.

6. Pulmonary Angiography

Pulmonary angiography was historically considered the gold standard for PE diagnosis, with high sensitivity and specificity. However, due to significant logistical challenges, technical difficulty, and potential complications (including up to 0.3% mortality), it is rarely used today.

7. Further Investigation of Isolated Subsegmental Pulmonary Embolism (SSPE)

Isolated SSPEs may be falsely positive in imaging studies. Additional tests are recommended, including:

Independent review by an experienced radiologist.

Leg imaging if not previously performed.

Alternative imaging tests for confirmation, when feasible.

Careful review by senior clinicians, considering the patient's medical history, comorbidities, and clinical condition.
False positives are common in isolated SSPE, and some guidelines allow for non-treatment of well-assessed low-risk patients with negative leg ultrasound.

Risk Stratification and Management of PE:

Upon diagnosing PE, patients should be risk-stratified to guide treatment decisions. Risk factors influencing prognosis include hemodynamic instability (e.g., hypotension or shock), syncope, prolonged respiratory failure, right ventricular (RV) strain, and significant underlying comorbidities.

1. Prognostic Indicators

In stable patients without overt shock, the prognosis may be assessed using the following indicators:

Historical Features: Such as syncope, collapse, or advanced age (>80 years).

Physical Examination: Findings of poor perfusion, borderline blood pressure, or new-onset atrial fibrillation.

Laboratory Investigations: Elevated troponin (especially if above myocardial infarction thresholds), elevated BNP, persistent lactate levels, and hypoxia.

Echocardiography or CTPA: Evidence of RV strain (e.g., RV/LV ratio >1.0), ventricular bowing, or RV dysfunction, with a mortality rate of 5% to 15%.
If these factors indicate severe PE, intensive management is required, which may include thrombolytic therapy.

2. Prognostic Scores
Various clinical scoring systems, such as the SPESI score, have been validated to identify low-risk PE patients suitable for home therapy. A high SPESI score is associated with poor prognosis, and patients with scores exceeding 15% mortality are considered high-risk.

Treatment:

1. General Measures

All PE patients should receive supportive care, including oxygen therapy, analgesia, and gentle fluid resuscitation (e.g., 250-mL boluses). Careful observation is necessary while determining the prognosis and initiating anticoagulation with direct oral anticoagulants (DOACs), low-molecular-weight heparin (LMWH), or fondaparinux unless contraindicated.

2. Heparin Therapy

While unfractionated heparin is considered less effective than LMWH, it remains useful for patients with severe renal dysfunction or those requiring thrombolysis.

3. Warfarin Therapy

If used, warfarin should be initiated alongside heparin and maintained for at least three months. The duration may be extended in patients at high risk, such as those with cancer or unprovoked large PE.

4. Direct Oral Anticoagulants (DOACs)

DOACs, including rivaroxaban, apixaban, and dabigatran, are increasingly favored due to their ease of use and fewer monitoring requirements compared to warfarin. Dosing adjustments may be necessary for patients with renal dysfunction or the elderly.

5. Caval Interruption Techniques

The use of caval interruption techniques is considered in patients with contraindications to anticoagulation or in those with recurrent PE despite appropriate therapy.

References

1. ESC Guidelines for the Diagnosis and Management of Acute Pulmonary Embolism. Eur Heart J. 2014. Oxford Academic. Available at:

https://academic.oup.com/eurheartj/article/35/43/3033/503581. Accessed February 2, 2018.

2. Kan Y, Yuan L, Meeks JK, et al. A meta-analysis on the accuracy of V/Q SPECT for diagnosing pulmonary embolism. Acta Radiol. 2015;56(5):565–572.

3. Kearon C, Akl EA, Ornelas J, et al. Antithrombotic Therapy for VTE Disease: CHEST Guideline and Expert Panel Report. Chest. 2016;149(2):315–352.

4. Kohn CG, Mearns ES, Parker MW, et al. Prognostic accuracy of clinical prediction rules for early all-cause mortality following pulmonary embolism: A bivariate meta-analysis. Chest. 2015;147(4):1043–1062.

5. Mountain D, Keijzers G, Chu K, et al. RESPECT-ED: Rates of Pulmonary Emboli (PE) and Subsegmental PE with Modern CT Pulmonary Angiograms in Emergency Departments. A multi-center observational study

demonstrating significant yield variation, uncorrelated with PE use or small PE rates. PLOS ONE. 2016;11(12):e0166483.

6. PIOPED Investigators. The Diagnostic Value of Ventilation/Perfusion Scans in Acute Pulmonary Embolism. Results from the Prospective Investigation of Pulmonary Embolism Diagnosis (PIOPED). JAMA. 1990;263(20):2753–2759.

7. Schouten HJ, Geersing GJ, Koek HL, et al. Diagnostic Accuracy of Conventional and Age-adjusted D-dimer Cutoff Values in Older Patients with Suspected Venous Thromboembolism: A Systematic Review and Meta-analysis. BMJ. 2013;346:f2492.

8. Roy PM, Colombet I, Durieux P, et al. Systematic Review and Meta-analysis of Strategies for Diagnosing Suspected Pulmonary Embolism. Br Med J. 2005;331:259.

9. Singh B, Mommer SK, Erwin PJ. Pulmonary Embolism Rule-out Criteria (PERC) in Pulmonary Embolism – Revisited: A Systematic Review and Meta-analysis. Emerg Med J. 2012;30(9):701–706.

10. Squizzato A, Donadini MP, Galli L. Prognostic Clinical Prediction Rules for Identifying Low-risk Pulmonary Embolism: A Systematic Review and Meta-analysis. J Thromb Haemost. 2012;10:1276–1290.

Chapter 6
Pericarditis, Cardiac Tamponade, and Myocarditis

Essentials

1. Myocarditis is frequently found in conjunction with pericarditis, which has significant clinical implications.

2. The diagnosis of pericarditis relies on patient history, electrocardiographic (ECG) findings, and echocardiographic results.

3. The majority of pericarditis cases are of idiopathic or viral origin and typically have a favorable prognosis.

4. Comprehensive evaluation of pericardial diseases requires multimodal imaging techniques.

5. Differentiating pericarditis from ST-segment elevation myocardial infarction (STEMI) is crucial. Administering fibrinolysis in pericarditis can lead to life-threatening complications, delay reperfusion therapy, and negatively affect patient outcomes.

6. Long-term monitoring is necessary, as some cases of pericarditis may progress to a subacute or chronic form, potentially resulting in complications such as chronic constrictive pericarditis.

Introduction

Pericarditis refers to the inflammation of the pericardium and can present as acute, sub-acute, or chronic, depending on the duration of symptoms and their recurrence. In many cases, pericarditis is accompanied by varying degrees of 'epi myocarditis,' making the term pericarditis more accurate. This condition most commonly affects young and middle-aged individuals, and it is more frequent in men than in women. Pericarditis has a low overall mortality rate of approximately 1.1%. The causes of pericarditis are listed in Table 5.6.2.

Clinical Features

History

Chest pain is the most common symptom, occurring in over 85-90% of cases. The pain is typically sharp and localized to the precordial or retrosternal area. It worsens during inspiration and tends to be positional, often alleviating when the patient sits up and leans forward. The pain may radiate to the trapezius ridge, neck, or shoulder, due to involvement of the phrenic nerve. The condition is often idiopathic, but a thorough history should investigate other potential causes, such as post-cardiac injury syndromes, rheumatologic diseases like systemic lupus erythematosus, and complications related to malignancies. Dyspnea is not a common symptom unless complications, such as cardiac tamponade or constrictive pericarditis, occur.

Examination

A detailed history and physical examination are essential in suspected pericarditis cases. Fever over 38°C is uncommon and may indicate bacterial (purulent) pericarditis. Sinus tachycardia is frequent, and a pericardial friction rub can be heard when the stethoscope is placed over the lower left sternal border, with the patient in the left lateral decubitus position. The rub is characterized by a superficial scratching or 'Velcro-like' sound. However, it can be transient or migratory, making it difficult to detect. Other signs like raised jugular venous pressure (JVP), hypotension, and may suggest cardiac tamponade, a potentially life-threatening complication present in up to 15% of acute idiopathic pericarditis cases.

High-Risk Features

Certain clinical signs should raise concern for serious underlying conditions such as tuberculosis (TB), bacterial infections, malignancy, or autoimmune diseases. These include:

Fever

Significant dyspnea

Sub-acute disease course

Large pericardial effusion or tamponade

Lack of response to aspirin or NSAIDs

History of anticoagulant use, immunosuppression, or recent trauma

Patients with suspected myocarditis, indicated by arrhythmias, significant ST-segment elevation, or elevated troponin levels

Clinical Investigations

Blood Tests

Full Blood Count: Leukocytosis is common, but significantly elevated white blood cell count may suggest bacterial infection.

Inflammatory Markers: The erythrocyte sedimentation rate (ESR) and C-reactive protein (CRP) levels help confirm inflammation and can monitor disease progression.

Troponin: A mild elevation in troponin levels may occur in acute pericarditis, but significant or sustained increases suggest concurrent myocarditis.

Chest X-ray

A chest X-ray is typically normal in acute pericarditis unless a large pericardial effusion is present. It is recommended by the European

Society of Cardiology (ESC) guidelines as part of the assessment for pericardial disease.

Electrocardiogram (ECG)

ECG is an essential diagnostic tool, showing abnormalities in approximately 90% of acute pericarditis cases, mainly due to the associated epi myocarditis. In rare "pure" cases of pericarditis, the ECG may be normal. The ECG progression is typically divided into four stages:

1. Stage 1: Widespread concave upward ST-segment elevation, PR depression, and the "Spodick sign" (down-sloping TP segments), seen in 60-80% of cases.

2. Stage 2: Normalization of PR and ST segments, sometimes transiently appearing normal.

3. Stage 3: T-wave inversion, typically occurring days to weeks after symptom onset.

4. Stage 4: Complete normalization of the ECG over up to 3 months, although T-wave changes may persist in some cases.

Echocardiography

Routine transthoracic echocardiography (TTE) is recommended in all acute pericarditis patients to detect pericardial fluid and assess its hemodynamic effects. It is especially useful when cardiac tamponade or constrictive pericarditis is suspected, and it helps differentiate pericarditis from acute myocardial infarction. TTE may not rule out pericarditis, but transesophageal echocardiography (TOE) offers better sensitivity for measuring pericardial thickness.

Advanced Imaging: CT/MRI

For cases with suspected malignancy, tuberculosis, or systemic inflammatory disorders, further imaging with computed tomography (CT) or magnetic resonance imaging (MRI) may be beneficial. These methods provide excellent views of the pericardium, identifying effusion, thickening, and lesions. MRI is particularly helpful in detecting late gadolinium enhancement in myopericarditis. FDG-PET/CT can reveal pericardial involvement in malignancy or tuberculosis.

Pericardiocentesis and Biopsy

In rare cases, pericardiocentesis and biopsy may be required for suspected bacterial, tuberculous, or neoplastic pericarditis, or in cases with cardiac tamponade, chronicity, or recurrence.

Diagnosis

The diagnosis of pericarditis is based on the presence of two or more of the following four criteria as outlined in the ESC guidelines:

1. Typical clinical history

2. Pericardial friction rub

3. Characteristic ECG changes

4. Pericardial effusion

Careful consideration should be given to differentiating pericarditis from other conditions such as pulmonary embolism, pneumothorax, and myocardial infarction, especially when using ECG features to distinguish between these conditions

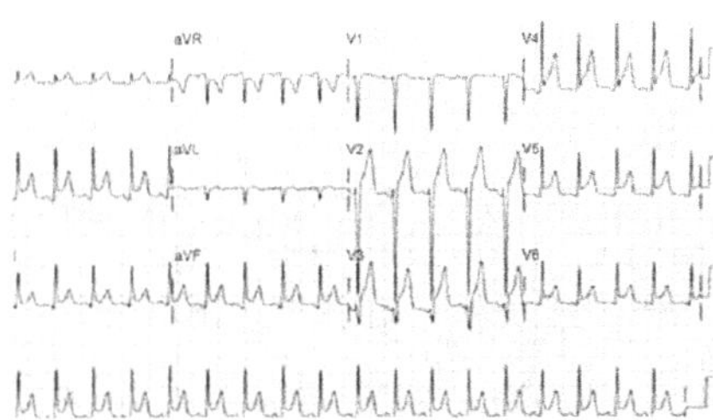

FIG. 5.6.1 Typical Electrocardiogram in pericarditis.

Classification of Pericarditis

The ESC Task Force classifies pericarditis into three categories:

1. Acute: Newly diagnosed pericarditis

2. Incessant: Pericarditis with persistent symptoms without clear remission after the acute episode

3. Chronic: Pericarditis lasting more than 3 months, with symptoms persisting beyond the typical duration of treatment.

Clinical Management and Treatment

In many cases, it is not necessary to identify the etiology of pericarditis, especially in areas with a low prevalence of tuberculosis. The focus is on managing the disease's symptoms, particularly in low-risk cases. High-risk features such as fever, large pericardial effusion, or failure to respond to

NSAIDs warrant hospitalization for further investigation and monitoring. Patients without high-risk features can typically be managed in an outpatient setting with close follow-up.

For patients with high-risk features, prompt intervention and close monitoring are critical to prevent complications, such as cardiac tamponade or persistent inflammation, which may require more aggressive treatment, including corticosteroids or immunosuppressive therapy.

Non-Steroidal Anti-Inflammatory Drugs (NSAIDs) in Acute Pericarditis

The primary objectives of treating acute pericarditis are to relieve symptoms, reduce inflammation, and prevent recurrence. NSAIDs, such as aspirin and ibuprofen, are commonly employed as first-line therapy. According to the ESC 2015 guidelines, these medications are the cornerstone of treatment. The duration of treatment should be based on symptom resolution and normalization of inflammatory markers, such as C-reactive protein (CRP). Studies involving several cohorts, including one randomized cohort study, indicate that NSAIDs are effective in about 70-80% of cases of viral or idiopathic pericarditis. In cases where patients do not respond or show worsening symptoms, further evaluation for other causes is necessary.

For aspirin, the recommended dosage is 750-1000 mg every 8 hours for the first 1-2 weeks, gradually reducing the dose by 250-500 mg every 1-2 weeks. For ibuprofen, the recommended dose is 600 mg every 8 hours for 1-2 weeks, followed by a reduction of 200-400 mg every 1-2 weeks. In patients with a history of acute myocardial infarction and pericarditis, aspirin is preferred due to the potential negative impact of NSAIDs on myocardial healing and scar formation.

Colchicine in Acute Pericarditis

Colchicine plays a crucial role in the treatment of acute pericarditis, not only by alleviating symptoms but also by reducing recurrence rates by approximately 50%. It should be administered alongside NSAIDs or aspirin. The ESC 2015 guidelines suggest administering 0.5 mg of colchicine daily for patients weighing less than 70 kg, or 0.5 mg twice daily for patients weighing more than 70 kg, for a duration of 3 months. The initial dose should be maintained until symptom resolution and normalization of biomarkers, after which a tapering schedule can be considered.

Corticosteroids in Acute Pericarditis

Although corticosteroids can be effective in treating acute pericarditis, their use is generally avoided as first-line therapy due to concerns about increased recurrence rates. The ESC guidelines recommend corticosteroids as a second-line option in patients who do not respond to NSAIDs and colchicine, and in those with specific underlying causes of pericarditis that require different treatments. In certain cases, such as systemic inflammatory diseases or uremia, or when NSAIDs are contraindicated, corticosteroids may be used as first-line therapy in conjunction with colchicine. The recommended dose of prednisone is between 0.2 and 0.5 mg/kg per day. Once symptoms resolve and CRP normalizes, the dose should be reduced gradually.

Management of Pericarditis in Pregnancy

For pregnant women with idiopathic pericarditis, corticosteroids are preferred, especially in the third trimester when NSAIDs are contraindicated due to the risk of premature closure of the ductus arteriosus. Colchicine is also contraindicated during pregnancy because of potential teratogenic effects.

Cardiac Tamponade: Non-Traumatic Case Management

Cardiac tamponade is a critical condition that results from the accumulation of fluid in the pericardial sac, leading to impaired heart function and potentially shock. Diagnosis is confirmed with echocardiography, which is also helpful in identifying early stages of tamponade. Treatment depends on the underlying cause and the rate of fluid accumulation. The priority is to drain the excess pericardial fluid. In certain cases, such as myocardial rupture or aortic dissection, thoracotomy with definitive repair is the preferred management approach, as pericardiocentesis may be harmful.

Clinical Features of Cardiac Tamponade

Cardiac tamponade symptoms can be nonspecific and vary depending on the speed and volume of fluid accumulation. The most common symptom is dyspnea, which is seen in 87-89% of cases. Other symptoms may include dizziness, faintness, and anxiety. On physical examination, signs such as hypotension, diminished heart sounds, and elevated jugular venous pressure (JVP) are commonly noted, though they may not always be present. Pulsus , tachycardia, and elevated JVP are also important clinical indicators.

Investigations for Cardiac Tamponade

Chest X-rays can show cardiomegaly in subacute or chronic cases, but this is a nonspecific finding. A more accurate diagnostic method is echocardiography, which is highly sensitive and specific for detecting pericardial effusion and tamponade. Transthoracic echocardiography (TTE) is typically the first choice, but transesophageal echocardiography (TOE) may be used if TTE is not feasible or yields inconclusive results. In some cases, computed tomography (CT) or magnetic resonance imaging (MRI) may be helpful if echocardiography is unavailable.

Treatment of Cardiac Tamponade

The mainstay of treatment for cardiac tamponade is the drainage of pericardial fluid. Pericardiocentesis, typically guided by ultrasound or fluoroscopy, is the preferred method for fluid drainage. In cases of purulent or recurrent effusions, or when tissue biopsy is required for diagnosis, surgical drainage may be necessary. Inotropic agents are generally ineffective, and mechanical ventilation should be avoided as it can worsen the condition by increasing intrathoracic pressure and decreasing cardiac output.

In summary, acute pericarditis and cardiac tamponade require prompt diagnosis and appropriate management, including the use of NSAIDs, colchicine, corticosteroids, and, in severe cases, pericardiocentesis or surgical drainage. The treatment strategy should be tailored to the patient's individual clinical situation, with a focus on relieving symptoms, preventing recurrence, and managing complications.

Myocarditis

Introduction

Myocarditis is defined by the World Health Organization (WHO) as an inflammatory condition of the myocardium, diagnosed using established histological, immunological, and immunohistochemical criteria. Often associated with pericarditis, it can result in a condition known as myopericarditis. The prognosis of myocarditis is highly dependent on the underlying cause. While treatment for many forms is symptomatic, the use of immune, histochemical, and molecular analyses of endomyocardial biopsy (EMB) along with autoantibody serum testing is essential for identifying patients who may benefit from targeted therapies.

Pathogenesis and Pathophysiology

Myocarditis can be triggered by a broad spectrum of viral, fungal, bacterial, protozoal, and parasitic infections, as well as toxins, medications, and immune-mediated diseases. The most frequent causes are listed in Table 5.6.4. Molecular techniques, particularly reverse transcriptase-polymerase chain reaction (RT-PCR), indicate that viral infections are the predominant cause of myocarditis. The precise mechanisms behind viral myocarditis and its long-term complications remain unclear, but it is believed to involve a combination of viral direct damage, immune system responses, and genetic predisposition.

Epidemiology

Due to its variable clinical presentation, the true incidence of myocarditis is not well understood. However, it is estimated to account for up to one-third of cases of dilated cardiomyopathy (DCM).

Clinical Features

The clinical manifestations of myocarditis can range from asymptomatic to severe. Possible presentations include:

Asymptomatic or subclinical

Fever with minimal cardiac symptoms, often associated with viral illnesses

Acute myopericarditis

Unexplained arrhythmias, including conduction delays

Unexplained cardiac failure, which can range from mild to cardiogenic shock

Sudden unexpected cardiac death

Delayed (years later) development of DCM

History

Many cases of myocarditis are asymptomatic, with symptoms often emerging 10 to 14 days after an antecedent viral infection. Patients may present with arrhythmias (e.g., palpitations or dizziness) or cardiac failure (e.g., shortness of breath). Associated pleuritic pain may occur due to concurrent pericarditis. In some cases, myocarditis may resemble an acute myocardial infarction (MI), with chest pain, ischemic changes on the ECG, and elevated cardiac biomarkers, especially in younger patients with no major cardiac risk factors and normal coronary angiograms.

Examination

Patients may present with a fever, though many remain infertile. Sinus tachycardia is common and may be disproportionate to the fever. Other arrhythmias, including conduction abnormalities, may be observed. A pericardial rub might be present if pericarditis is also present. Signs of heart failure can range from mild symptoms to severe pulmonary edema or cardiogenic shock.

First-Line Clinical Investigations

Diagnosing acute viral myocarditis in the emergency department (ED) typically relies on presumptive diagnosis, as definitive diagnosis requires specialized tests. Clinicians should consider myocarditis in patients, particularly younger individuals, who present with unexplained cardiac failure, shock, or arrhythmias. Initial testing can provide supportive evidence for the diagnosis.

Disposition

Pericardial effusion, if left untreated, can lead to cardiac tamponade, which can be fatal if not managed promptly. The rate of fluid accumulation, the compliance of the pericardium, and the volume of fluid influence the rapidity of onset. Patients with clinically compensated non-traumatic cardiac tamponade should be closely monitored for potential drainage under image-guided techniques.

Controversies

Key issues in myocarditis management include:

Distinguishing between clinical and echocardiographic tamponade, especially with advancements in imaging technology.

Determining the appropriate type and timing of drainage procedures in critically ill patients.

Common Causes of Myocarditis

More frequent causes of myocarditis include various viruses (e.g., adenovirus, coxsackie B virus), toxins (e.g., anthracyclines, ethanol), and immune-mediated conditions (e.g., Chagas disease, systemic lupus erythematosus).

Essentials

1. Myocarditis is most commonly caused by viral infections and typically has a favorable prognosis, with many patients recovering fully.

2. Acute, fulminant myocarditis can present with life-threatening arrhythmias or cardiac failure, but patients may recover fully with supportive care.

3. Myocarditis can mimic myocardial infarction with chest pain, ECG changes, and elevated cardiac biomarkers.

4. Long-term follow-up is essential for patients who have experienced myocarditis to monitor for potential development of DCM.

Laboratory Tests

Laboratory tests can provide supporting evidence for myocarditis diagnosis. Elevated white blood cell count, erythrocyte sedimentation rate (ESR), and C-reactive protein (CRP) levels, along with cardiac biomarkers like troponin and brain natriuretic peptide (BNP), are commonly observed. These parameters can also assist in evaluating treatment responses.

Chest X-ray

In severe cases, chest x-rays may show cardiomegaly and signs of congestive heart failure. However, a normal chest x-ray is also possible.

Electrocardiography (ECG)

Most patients with myocarditis will have an abnormal ECG, but the changes are nonspecific. The most common findings include sinus tachycardia and non-specific ST-T wave changes. ST elevation may be seen, but it typically appears concave and diffuse without reciprocal changes. Arrhythmias, including conduction delays, may also be present.

Echocardiography

Echocardiography provides supportive evidence but is not diagnostic for myocarditis. Global or regional wall motion abnormalities and associated pericardial effusion may be seen. Signs of myocardial failure, such as ventricular dilation and reduced ejection fraction, may also be present.

Cardiac Magnetic Resonance Imaging (MRI) and Electrocardiography-Gated Multidetector CT

Cardiac MRI has become increasingly useful for diagnosing myocarditis and tracking disease progression. It correlates well with areas of myocarditis, revealing abnormal signal regions. MRI can also assist in identifying biopsy targets. Electrocardiography-gated CT is likely to show myocardial hyper-enhancement patterns indicative of myocarditis.

Coronary Angiography

Coronary angiography is often necessary to exclude significant coronary artery disease, especially in patients who present with chest pain similar to that of a myocardial infarction.

Endomyocardial Biopsy (EMB)

Currently, EMB is the gold standard for definitive diagnosis of myocarditis. However, there are several challenges with this approach:

Acute myocarditis can be patchy, and a single biopsy may miss the diagnosis.

False positives can occur.

It may overestimate the severity of the condition in less severe cases.

Despite controversies regarding patient selection for EMB, it remains the definitive diagnostic tool, though complications such as venous injury, arrhythmias, and cardiac perforation can occur.

Treatment and Disposition

Treatment primarily focuses on managing heart failure and providing supportive care, which may progress to the use of implantable defibrillators or mechanical assist devices as a bridge to heart transplantation. In cases of pulmonary edema, ventilatory support is essential. Diuretics, vasodilators, and inotropes are used to optimize cardiac output and filling. Angiotensin-converting enzyme inhibitors (ACEIs) and angiotensin II receptor blockers (ARBs) should be started early. Anti-arrhythmic treatments are applied to manage complications. For patients who progress to cardiogenic shock, early and aggressive intervention is required, potentially including extracorporeal membrane oxygenation (ECMO) or ventricular assist devices as a bridge to recovery or transplant. Immunosuppressive therapy has shown limited success, with no trials proving significant clinical benefit. However, preliminary data on interferon-β therapy for patients with viral genome detection are promising, though further multicenter studies are needed.

Controversies

The effectiveness and appropriate use of interferon, immunoglobulin, and corticosteroids in the treatment of viral myocarditis.

The ideal diagnostic approach for myocarditis, particularly in determining the role of MRI in its identification.

The utility of endomyocardial biopsy (EMB) in patients suspected of having myocarditis due to autoimmune conditions

Prognosis

The prognosis of acute myocarditis is largely determined by the severity of symptoms, histological findings, and biomarkers. Key predictors of a poor prognosis include hypotension, elevated pulmonary wedge pressure, and biochemical markers such as elevated Fas, anti-myosin autoantibodies, and IL-10. Increased tumor necrosis factor-α and persistent viral genome expression are also associated with poor recovery. While many cases of myocarditis resolve without long-term complications, some progress to chronic dilated cardiomyopathy or recurrent arrhythmias. In severe cases, sudden cardiac death may occur, particularly in younger individuals.

References

1. ESC Guidelines on the diagnosis and management of acute pulmonary embolism. Eur Heart J. 2014. Oxford Academic. Available at: https://academic.oup.com/eurheartj/article/35/43/3033/503581. Accessed February 2, 2018.

2. Kan Y, Yuan L, Meeks JK, et al. The accuracy of V/Q SPECT in the diagnosis of pulmonary embolism: a meta-analysis. Acta Radiol. 2015;56(5):565-572.

3. Kearon C, Akl EA, Ornelas J, et al. Antithrombotic therapy for VTE disease: CHEST Guideline and Expert Panel Report. Chest. 2016;149(2):315-352.

4. Kohn CG, Mearns ES, Parker MW, et al. Prognostic accuracy of clinical prediction rules for early post-pulmonary embolism all-cause mortality: a bivariate meta-analysis. Chest. 2015;147(4):1043-1062.

5. Mountain D, Keijzers G, Chu K, et al. RESPECT-ED: Rates of pulmonary emboli and subsegmental PE with modern CT pulmonary angiograms in emergency departments: A multi-center observational study. PLOS ONE. 2016;11(12):e0166483.

6. PIOPED Investigators. Value of the ventilation/perfusion scan in acute pulmonary embolism: Results of the PIOPED study. JAMA. 1990;263(20):2753-2759.

7. Schouten HJ, Geersing GJ, Koek HL, et al. Diagnostic accuracy of conventional or age-adjusted D-dimer cut-off values in older patients with suspected venous thromboembolism: A systematic review and meta-analysis. BMJ. 2013;346:f2492.

8. Roy PM, Colombet I, Durieux P, et al. Systematic review and meta-analysis of strategies for diagnosing suspected pulmonary embolism. Br Med J. 2005;331:259.

9. Singh B, Mommer SK, Erwin PJ. Pulmonary embolism rule-out criteria (PERC) revisited: A systematic review and meta-analysis. Emerg Med J. 2012;30(9):701-706.

10. Squizzato A, Donadini MP, Galli L. Prognostic clinical prediction rules to identify

low-risk pulmonary embolism: A systematic review and meta-analysis. J Thromb Haemost. 2012;10:1276-1290.

11. Adler Y, Charron P, Imazio M, et al. 2015 ESC guidelines for the diagnosis and management of pericardial diseases: Task force for the diagnosis and management of pericardial diseases of the European Society of Cardiology, endorsed by the European Association for Cardio-Thoracic Surgery. Eur Heart J. 2015;36(42):2921-2964.

12. Celik T, Ozturk C, Balta S, Iyisoy A. The role of combined electrocardiogram criteria in the differential diagnosis of acute pericarditis: PR segment and QT interval. Am J Emerg Med. 2016;34(7):1309.

13. Chhabra L, Spodick DH. Ideal isoelectric reference segment in pericarditis: A suggested approach to a commonly prevailing clinical misconception. Cardiology. 2012;122(4):210-212.

14. Cosyns B, Plein S, Nihoyannopoulos P, et al. European Association of Cardiovascular Imaging (EACVI) position paper: Multimodality imaging in pericardial disease. Eur Heart J Cardiovasc Imaging. 2015;16(1):12-31.

15. Imazio M, Belli R, Brucato A, et al. Rationale and design of the COlchicine for Prevention of the Post-pericardiotomy Syndrome and Post-operative Atrial Fibrillation (COPPS-2 trial): A randomized, placebo-controlled, multicenter study on the use of colchicine for the primary prevention of the postpericardiotomy syndrome, postoperative effusions, and postoperative atrial fibrillation. Am Heart J. 2013;166(1):13-19.

16. Imazio M, Lazaros G, Brucato A, Gaita F. Recurrent pericarditis: New and emerging therapeutic options. Nat Rev Cardiol. 2016;13(2):99-105.

17. McCanny P, Colreavy F. Echocardiographic approach to cardiac tamponade in critically ill patients. J Crit Care. 2017;39:271-277.

18. Inglis R, King AJ, Gleave M, et al. Pericardiocentesis in contemporary practice. J Invasive Cardiol. 2011;23(6):234-239.

19. Maggiolini S, Gentile G, Farina A, et al. Safety, efficacy, and complications of pericardiocentesis by real-time echo-monitored procedure. Am J Cardiol. 2016;117(8):1369-1374.

20. Caforio AL, Pankuweit S, Arbustini E, et al. Current state of knowledge on etiology, diagnosis, management, and therapy of myocarditis: A position statement of the European Society of Cardiology Working Group on Myocardial and Pericardial Diseases. Eur Heart J. 2013;34(33):2636-2651.

Chapter 7
Heart Valve Emergencies: Overview and Clinical Management

Heart valve emergencies are critical events that can lead to sudden and severe deterioration in cardiac function. The underlying pathology varies depending on which valve is affected, with infective endocarditis being a key culprit.

Infective Endocarditis: A Frequently Overlooked Diagnosis

Infective endocarditis (IE) is often misdiagnosed, highlighting the need for a high level of clinical suspicion. A delay in diagnosis can significantly increase both morbidity and mortality rates.

Epidemiology

Infective endocarditis occurs at a rate of 3 to 10 cases per 100,000 person-years, with prosthetic valve endocarditis (PVE) accounting for 20% to 30% of these cases. The condition predominantly affects males (with a male-to-female ratio of ≥2:1) and is most commonly seen in individuals aged 50 to 60.

In developing countries, rheumatic heart disease remains the most common risk factor for IE, while in developed countries, the risk factors have shifted. These include:

Host-related factors: Poor oral hygiene, intravenous drug use (IVDU), severe renal disease requiring hemodialysis, diabetes, mitral valve prolapse (especially with valve incompetence), and degenerative valve changes.

Procedure-related factors: Infections associated with intravascular devices, genitourinary and gastrointestinal procedures, or surgical wound infections.

Pathophysiology of Infective Endocarditis

Infective endocarditis involves a complex interaction between the host and pathogens. Platelet-fibrin deposits form on sites of endothelial injury, which become infected and lead to the formation of vegetations. These vegetations can embolize, causing septic emboli and subsequent tissue ischemia. The local destruction of the valve may result in further complications, such as rupture of chordae , abscess formation, and conduction abnormalities.

Changing Microbial Landscape in Infective Endocarditis

Staphylococcus aureus has emerged as the most common pathogen in both native and prosthetic valve endocarditis, overtaking Streptococcus viridans. This shift reflects improvements in dental hygiene and an increase in nosocomial infections. Approximately 13% to 25% of patients with S. aureus bacteremia develop infective endocarditis.

Nosocomial endocarditis occurs after 72 hours of hospital admission or within 4 to 8 weeks of invasive procedures, with S. aureus and Enterococcus species being the most common causative organisms. Fungal infections, accounting for less than 10% of cases, are more common in individuals with IVDU, immunocompromised patients, or those with prosthetic valves.

Prevention and Prophylaxis

Prophylactic antibiotic administration before procedures is an important preventive measure, particularly for high-risk patients. High-risk patients include those with prosthetic heart valves, significant mitral valve prolapse, and those with congenital or acquired valve dysfunction. However, recent guidelines have reduced the need for prophylaxis in many cases, including gastrointestinal and genitourinary procedures. Dental procedures that involve manipulation of the gingival tissue or periapical regions may still warrant prophylaxis for high-risk individuals.

Recommended prophylaxis includes a single-dose antibiotic, administered 30 to 60 minutes before the procedure. Options include amoxicillin or ampicillin for non-penicillin allergic patients, or clindamycin for those with allergies.

Clinical Features of Infective Endocarditis

Infective endocarditis should be recognized as a multisystem disease with nonspecific symptoms. The most common signs include fever (80% to 85% of cases), malaise (up to 95%), and potentially unexplained systemic symptoms such as headache, cough, chest pain, dyspnea, and weight loss. Importantly, fever may be absent in severely debilitated or elderly patients, or those on antibiotics.

Clinical examination may reveal a new or altered heart murmur, though many patients already have a murmur present. Additionally, petechiae, splinter hemorrhages, Osler nodes, Janeway lesions, and Roth spots can occur due to systemic embolization. A new or changed murmur is a particularly significant finding, especially in those with prosthetic valves or congestive heart failure.

Complications of Infective Endocarditis

Cardiac Complications:

Congestive heart failure (CHF): This occurs due to valvular damage, particularly if the aortic valve is involved.

Conduction abnormalities: These may result from extension of the infection into the conduction system, including atrioventricular blocks or bundle-branch blocks.

Pericarditis and tamponade: Rare but possible if the infection extends to the sinus of Valsalva.

Myocardial infarction: This can occur when septic emboli block coronary arteries, though it is uncommon.

Neurological Complications: Neurological manifestations occur in approximately 15% of cases, usually due to embolism from left-sided valve lesions. These include stroke, transient ischemic attacks, and meningoencephalitis, with a high mortality rate.

Systemic Embolization: Systemic emboli can affect any organ, though splenic, hepatic, and renal emboli are most common. In right-sided endocarditis, especially involving the tricuspid valve, pulmonary emboli and abscesses are typical.

Renal Dysfunction: This may result from immune complex-mediated glomerulonephritis, altered renal hemodynamics, or nephrotoxicity due to antibiotics or other treatments.

Clinical Presentation and Diagnosis of Infective Endocarditis

Clinical Presentation

Infective endocarditis (IE) is often indicated by persistent bacteremia or fever, despite treatment, along with congestive heart failure (CHF) or the emergence of new ECG features, such as atrioventricular heart block, fascicular block, and bundle branch block. Early detection and clinical investigation are crucial for effective management.

Diagnostic Investigations

1. Blood Cultures: For stable patients without complications, three sets of blood cultures should be obtained from different vascular puncture sites, spaced at least an hour apart

within a 24-hour window, before initiating empirical antibiotics. Bacteremia is typically continuous, so the timing of venipuncture does not need to coincide with fever. Both aerobic and anaerobic media should be employed for each sample. In critically ill patients, blood culture timing can be reduced, as early antibiotic treatment should not be delayed.

2. Full Blood Count (FBC): Anemia, usually normochromic and normocytic, is common. Leukocytosis may be observed in acute infective endocarditis but is not always present in subacute cases. Thrombocytopenia is rare.

3. Inflammatory Markers:

Erythrocyte Sedimentation Rate (ESR): This non-specific test is elevated in nearly all patients with IE, often surpassing 55 mm/h. A normal ESR makes infective endocarditis less likely.

C-Reactive Protein (CRP): Another non-specific marker, CRP is typically more sensitive than ESR in diagnosing IE.

Procalcitonin: Although raised in IE cases, procalcitonin is less sensitive than CRP.

4. Urinalysis: Abnormal urinalysis is found in about 50% of cases, showing proteinuria and microscopic hematuria. However, renal function may remain normal.

5. Echocardiography: Echocardiography is essential for confirming the diagnosis by visualizing heart valves, assessing hemodynamic impact, and identifying complications like perivalvular involvement and abscesses. Transthoracic echocardiography (TTE) is the first-line imaging tool in suspected infective endocarditis and should be performed promptly. TTE's sensitivity for detecting vegetations is

70% for native valve endocarditis (NVE), but its specificity remains high at 95%. The sensitivity in prosthetic valve endocarditis (PVE) is lower at 50%. Transesophageal echocardiography (TOE), although more invasive, offers higher sensitivity (92-96%) and specificity (90%) for vegetations and can better identify perivalvular lesions and abscesses. It is recommended for cases with poor TTE quality or high clinical suspicion of IE despite negative TTE results.

Duke Criteria for Infective Endocarditis Diagnosis

The Duke Criteria is a set of guidelines to help diagnose infective endocarditis:

Major Criteria:

Positive blood cultures for typical IE organisms or persistently positive blood cultures.

Imaging evidence of IE, such as vegetations, abscesses, or valve perforations, confirmed by echocardiography or PET/CT.

Minor Criteria:

Predisposing conditions like heart disease or intravenous drug use.

Fever exceeding 38°C.

Vascular phenomena like major arterial emboli or septic pulmonary infarcts.

Immunological phenomena such as glomerulonephritis or Osler nodes.

Microbiological evidence from blood cultures or serological tests that are consistent with IE.

Treatment

Effective management of infective endocarditis requires a multifaceted approach:

1. Antibiotic Therapy: Empirical antibiotic treatment should be started immediately after blood cultures are taken, especially in critically ill patients. The goal is to eradicate the pathogen, but due to the difficulty of achieving effective drug levels within vegetations, long-term therapy (4 to 6 weeks) is usually necessary. Once the pathogen is identified, antibiotics are tailored accordingly. The ESC guidelines recommend a combination of ampicillin, flucloxacillin, and gentamicin for community-acquired NVE or late prosthetic valve endocarditis. For penicillin-allergic patients, vancomycin and gentamicin are used.

2. Surgical Intervention: Surgical management may be required if the patient is hemodynamically unstable or if there are complications such as heart failure, valve perforation, or abscess formation. Surgery may

also be indicated for larger vegetations or virulent organisms resistant to antibiotics.

3. Anticoagulation: The use of anticoagulants like aspirin or warfarin in infective endocarditis is not recommended, as it has not shown to reduce the risk of embolic events and may increase the risk of bleeding, especially intracranial bleeding. Anticoagulants should only be used if indicated for other conditions, such as the presence of a prosthetic valve.

Prognosis

The overall mortality for native and prosthetic valve endocarditis ranges from 20% to 25% at one year and increases to 50% at ten years. The most common causes of death are congestive heart failure, hemodynamic instability, and embolic complications. Mortality is higher in cases caused by resistant organisms like

Pseudomonas aeruginosa or fungal infections. The mortality rate in right-sided endocarditis among intravenous drug users is lower at 10%. Additionally, relapse rates vary by causative organisms, with S. aureus showing the highest relapse rate.

Acute Aortic Incompetence

Etiology and Pathophysiology: Acute aortic valve incompetence can be caused by infective endocarditis, aortic dissection, blunt trauma, or valve rupture. This condition leads to acute volume overload in the left ventricle, which results in increased left ventricular end-diastolic pressure. This pressure is transmitted to the left atrium and pulmonary venous system, causing pulmonary edema. Cardiac output decreases as blood is diverted into both the forward flow and regurgitant backflow into the left atrium.

Clinical Features: Patients with acute aortic incompetence typically present with severe congestive heart failure and hypotension. They may also report ischemic chest pain due to myocardial ischemia, even in the absence of coronary artery disease. Immediate management is critical to prevent hemodynamic collapse.

Mitral Stenosis: Pathophysiology, Acute Deterioration, and Treatment

Pathophysiology of Mitral Stenosis

The normal mitral valve area is between 4 to 6 cm^2 in adults. Symptom onset typically occurs when the valve orifice narrows to less than 2.5 cm^2, and severe stenosis is defined when the area is reduced to 1 cm^2. However, patients may remain asymptomatic for many years. As stenosis worsens, the left atrium faces an increased pressure load, leading to pulmonary congestion and the development of pulmonary hypertension.

The most common cause of mitral stenosis is rheumatic heart disease. Other less frequent causes include atrial myxomas, significant annular calcification, and ball-valve thrombi. Congenital causes are rare.

Pathophysiology of Acute Deterioration in Mitral Stenosis

Acute deterioration in mitral stenosis can be triggered in two main ways:

1. Increased Heart Rate: Elevated heart rate reduces ventricular filling time during diastole, leading to increased atrial pressure. This pressure is transmitted back to the pulmonary vascular bed, resulting in acute dyspnea and pulmonary edema. Atrial fibrillation with rapid ventricular response is a common cause of this phenomenon. The absence of atrial contraction in atrial fibrillation reduces cardiac output by about 20%, contributing to hemodynamic instability.

2. Increased Flow Across the Stenosed Valve: An increase in flow through the stenotic valve results in a higher pressure gradient, which is proportional to the square of the flow rate. This increase raises left atrial pressure, precipitating pulmonary congestion. Common situations where transvalvular flow increases include sepsis, physical exertion, pregnancy, hypervolemia, and hyperthyroidism.

Clinical Features of Mitral Stenosis

Patients may remain asymptomatic for a prolonged period, though physical examinations often reveal abnormalities. Once symptoms manifest, they typically include:

Dyspnea and Fatigue

Thromboembolic Events

Atrial Fibrillation

Pulmonary Congestion

As the disease progresses, signs of severe stenosis such as small pulse pressure, soft heart sounds, and signs of pulmonary hypertension (e.g., right ventricular heave and loud P2) become evident. Acute pulmonary edema and atrial fibrillation with a rapid ventricular rate are also common.

Auscultatory findings often include:

Loud First Heart Sound

Opening Snap

Mid-Diastolic Murmur with Presystolic Accentuation

Clinical Investigations

1. Chest X-Ray (CXR) and Electrocardiography (ECG):

CXR typically shows left atrial enlargement, pulmonary congestion, and pulmonary hypertension, with a normal heart size.

Left atrial enlargement is seen on ECG in about 90% of patients in sinus rhythm.

2. Echocardiography:

This is the primary diagnostic tool. It confirms the diagnosis, helps rule out other causes of mitral valve obstruction, and assesses the severity of stenosis and pulmonary artery pressure.

Treatment of Mitral Stenosis

Medical management focuses on symptom relief and preventing complications, but it does not halt the disease progression. Surgical intervention is the definitive treatment, typically when symptoms are severe, classified as New York Heart Association (NYHA) functional class III.

1. Medical Management:

Pulmonary Edema: Treated with diuretics or long-acting nitrates.

Atrial Fibrillation with Rapid Ventricular Response: Rate control is prioritized, using medications or cardioversion.

Anticoagulation: Indicated for patients with atrial fibrillation to prevent thromboembolism.

2. Surgical Treatment:

Percutaneous Mitral Balloon Valvotomy: Considered in patients with moderate or severe stenosis without left atrial thrombus or significant mitral regurgitation.

Mitral Valve Surgery: Surgical commissurotomy or valve replacement may be required in patients with unfavorable valve morphology or severe stenosis.

Prognosis

Asymptomatic or Minimally Symptomatic Patients: The 10-year survival rate is greater than 80%.

Symptomatic Patients: The 10-year survival rate drops to 0-15%.

Mortality: In untreated patients, death is often due to complications such as pulmonary congestion, right heart failure, systemic or pulmonary emboli, and infective endocarditis.

Acute Mitral Incompetence: Pathophysiology, Clinical Features, and Treatment

Pathophysiology of Acute Mitral Incompetence

In acute mitral incompetence, the volume overload in the left atrium due to regurgitation is the primary factor. The left atrium's limited capacity to accommodate the extra volume leads to pulmonary edema. Increased pulmonary vascular resistance and right ventricular failure can also occur. Cardiac output is reduced because of a lower stroke volume, and systemic vascular resistance further impedes output. Tachycardia often develops but provides no benefit due to reduced diastolic filling time.

Etiology of Acute Mitral Incompetence

The causes include:

Infective Endocarditis

Papillary Muscle Dysfunction

Myocardial Ischemia or Infarction

Trauma

Infiltrative Diseases

Chordae Tendineae Rupture

Acute Rheumatic Fever

Atrial Myxoma

Systemic Lupus Erythematosus

Clinical Features

Acute mitral valve incompetence presents acutely with:

Reduced Perfusion

Acute Pulmonary Edema

Variable Blood Pressure: Can be either normal or low.

Precordial Findings: May include a third heart sound, and a soft, early systolic mitral murmur that radiates to the axilla.

Clinical Investigations

1. Chest X-Ray (CXR): Shows pulmonary edema without cardiomegaly.

2. ECG: May show recent infarction if it was the precipitating factor.

3. Echocardiography: Essential for diagnosis, as it identifies the lesion and assesses left ventricular function. Both transthoracic echocardiography (TTE) and transesophageal

echocardiography (TOE) may be necessary for comprehensive assessment.

Treatment of Acute Mitral Incompetence

1. Medical Management: Primarily aimed at stabilizing the patient until surgery can be performed.

In normotensive patients, sodium nitroprusside may be used to reduce regurgitant volume and pulmonary congestion.

In hypotensive patients, a combination of sodium nitroprusside and an inotrope like dobutamine may be required.

Aortic Balloon Counterpulsation: This can assist in improving left ventricular ejection volume but does not significantly improve outcomes.

2. Surgical Management: Urgent surgery is often required, with valve repair preferred over replacement due to better outcomes.

Prognosis

Mortality: High in patients with severe left ventricular failure. Urgent surgical intervention is critical to improving survival chances.

References

1. Ambrosioni, J., Hernandez-Meneses, M., Téllez, A., et al. (2017). The evolving epidemiology of infective endocarditis in the twenty-first century. Current Infectious Disease Reports, 19, 21.

2. Bai, A.D., Steinberg, M., Showler, A., et al. (2017). Diagnostic accuracy of transthoracic echocardiography for detecting infective

endocarditis, using transesophageal echocardiography as the reference standard: A meta-analysis. Journal of the American Society of Echocardiography, 30(7), 639–646.

3. Baumgartner, H., Falk, V., Bax, J.J., et al. (2017). 2017 ESC/EACTS Guidelines for the management of valvular heart disease. European Heart Journal, 38(36), 2739–2791.

4. Habib, G., Lancellotti, P., Antunes, M.J., et al. (2015). 2015 ESC guidelines for the management of infective endocarditis: A task force from the European Society of Cardiology (ESC), endorsed by the European Association for Cardio-Thoracic Surgery (EACTS) and the European Association of Nuclear Medicine (EANM). European Heart Journal, 36(44), 3075–3128.

5. Kang, D.H., Kim, Y.J., Kim, S.H., et al. (2012). Early surgery versus conventional treatment for infective endocarditis. New

England Journal of Medicine, 366(26), 2466–2473.

6. Nishimura, R.A., Otto, C.M., Bonow, R.O., et al. (2017). 2017 AHA/ACC focused update of the 2014 AHA/ACC guideline for the management of patients with valvular heart disease: A report of the American College of Cardiology/American Heart Association Task Force on Clinical Practice Guidelines. Circulation, 135(25), e1159–e1195.

7. NICE Clinical Guidelines, No. 64. (2016). Prophylaxis Against Infective Endocarditis. National Institute for Health and Care Excellence (UK). Retrieved from http://www.nice.org.uk/CG064.

8. Sharma, V., Candilio, L., Hausenloy, D.J. (2012). Infective endocarditis: An intensive care perspective. Trends in Anaesthesia and Critical Care, 2(1), 36–41.

9. Thuny, F., Grisoli, D., Collart, F., et al. (2012). Management of infective endocarditis: Challenges and perspectives. The Lancet, 379(9819), 965–975.

10. Wang, A., Athan, E., Pappas, P.A., et al. (2012). Contemporary clinical profile and outcomes of prosthetic valve infective endocarditis. European Heart Journal, 33(16), 2019–2025.

Chapter 8
Peripheral Vascular Disease

Essentials

1. The prevalence of peripheral arterial and venous diseases is rising in developed countries, driven by the growing elderly population.

2. Claudication remains the primary symptom of arterial disease in the limbs, though well-developed collateral circulation can delay the onset of symptomatic limb ischemia.

3. Acute arterial occlusion is characterized by distinct symptoms and signs. It is a critical emergency that demands immediate intervention by a skilled vascular surgeon.

4. In cases of suspected venous thrombosis, thorough evaluation is crucial. Unfortunately, the presence or absence of deep venous thrombosis

(DVT) symptoms does not reliably indicate the presence of a venous clot.

5. The optimal approach to diagnosing DVT involves establishing a pre-test probability and conducting appropriate non-invasive tests initially.

6. Compression ultrasonography is considered the gold standard for diagnosing DVT.

7. Anticoagulation therapy is recommended for DVT located above the popliteal vein. Although the management of below-knee DVT remains debated, mounting evidence supports anticoagulation for these cases to prevent complications.

8. Extensive thrombus in the ilio-femoral region or the upper limb may necessitate early surgical intervention or thrombolytic therapy to reduce the risk of post-thrombotic syndrome.

Arterial Disease: Acute and Chronic Extremity Ischaemia

Ischaemia in the extremities can be classified as acute, chronic, or acute-on-chronic, with the severity and presentation influenced by the development of collateral circulation.

Chronic Arterial Ischaemia

Epidemiology, Pathogenesis, and Pathology: Peripheral arterial disease (PAD) becomes more prevalent with age, with most symptomatic patients being over 60. Between the ages of 50-70, men have a higher incidence, but after 70, the prevalence is nearly equal in both genders, at 15-20%. PAD is often caused by atherosclerosis affecting the lower abdominal aorta, iliac, femoral, and popliteal arteries. Contributing factors, such as diabetes mellitus, hypertension, smoking, hyperlipidaemia, and prior limb surgery, accelerate the progression of the disease. Over time, collateral circulation can develop as an adaptive response to arterial blockages. These pre-existing pathways from medium and large arteries increase blood flow to the affected area, but they may not fully meet the increased demands during physical exertion.

Clinical Features: Chronic ischaemia manifests as claudication, a cramping pain triggered by consistent physical activity and relieved by rest. The most common site of occlusion causing claudication is the superficial femoral artery, often resulting in calf pain. Less commonly, occlusions in the aortoiliac region can cause thigh or buttock pain. As ischaemia worsens, rest pain in the foot, exacerbated by elevation, may develop, signifying inadequate blood flow. Clinical examination may reveal absent or diminished distal pulses, bruits (especially in the femoral area), and signs of tissue ischaemia, such as pallor, atrophic skin changes, and non-healing ulcers or gangrene.

Clinical Investigations: Blood tests should assess renal and hepatic function, as well as exclude anemia, polycythaemia, hyperglycaemia, and hyperlipidaemia. In patients under 50, thrombophilia screening may be necessary. The ankle-brachial pressure index (ABPI) is crucial in confirming the diagnosis of PAD. A resting ABPI below 0.9 indicates arterial disease, with values between 0.5 and 0.9 associated with claudication and below 0.5 indicating rest pain. Duplex ultrasound is used for initial assessment, while computed tomography angiography (CTA) and magnetic resonance angiography (MRA) offer detailed, non-invasive imaging of the arterial tree.

Treatment: Management focuses on preventing disease progression. This includes regular exercise, smoking cessation, and controlling associated conditions such as diabetes, hypertension, and hyperlipidaemia. Low-dose aspirin is commonly used, but warfarin and dual antiplatelet therapy are generally not beneficial. Statins are recommended for all patients with PAD. For advanced disease, multidisciplinary vascular assessments are essential, and surgical or endovascular interventions may be considered to address complications like ulcers or gangrene.

Acute Arterial Ischaemia of the Lower Limb

Pathogenesis and Pathology: Acute lower limb ischaemia, or limb-threatening ischaemia, is associated with high morbidity and mortality. Causes include embolism (most commonly from the heart, especially in atrial fibrillation), thrombosis, trauma, or iatrogenic factors. Embolic events are the most common, with the majority originating from thrombi in the left atrium or atrial appendage.

Clinical Features: The sudden onset of arterial occlusion is a medical emergency. Classic signs include the "6 Ps": pulselessness, pain, pallor, paraesthesia, paralysis, and "perishing cold." These symptoms may evolve rapidly, with the limb becoming pale, cold, and eventually cyanotic as the ischaemia progresses. Pain is severe and unrelenting, requiring opioid analgesia for relief. If not treated within 6 hours, irreversible tissue damage, including gangrene, can occur.

Clinical Investigation: Doppler ultrasound is essential for assessing the arterial circulation and locating the site of occlusion. Basic blood tests, electrocardiography, and chest radiography help exclude other conditions and identify contributing factors, such as arrhythmias or low cardiac output.

Differential Diagnosis: Differentiating between embolism and thrombosis is crucial. Embolic events tend to cause rapid onset symptoms, whereas thrombosis develops more slowly in patients with pre-existing PAD and collateral circulation. Phlegmasia , a massive iliofemoral deep vein thrombosis (DVT), must also be considered, as it can present similarly, but typically causes marked swelling and a cyanotic limb, unlike the sharp demarcation seen with embolism.

Treatment: Early recognition and prompt intervention are critical. Revascularization should occur as soon as possible to restore blood flow. Intra-arterial heparin and opioid analgesia should be administered immediately. Revascularization options include thrombolytic therapy, mechanical thrombus extraction, or surgical thrombectomy. For patients with neurological deficits, thrombus extraction or surgical thrombectomy is preferred, while catheter-directed thrombolysis is suitable for less severe cases. Prompt treatment can prevent irreversible damage and improve limb salvage outcomes.

In cases where ischaemia lasts more than 14 days, advanced procedures such as bypass surgery may be required, depending on the cause and extent of the occlusion.

Outpatient treatment is typically preferred by patients due to its convenience and lower cost. However, hospitalization may be necessary for cases involving severe edema in the entire lower limb or thrombus extending above the groin.

An alternative to low-molecular-weight heparin (LMWH) and warfarin is the direct factor Xa inhibitor, rivaroxaban. Initially, rivaroxaban is administered at 15 mg twice daily for the first three weeks following diagnosis, then reduced to 20 mg once daily for the duration of treatment. It is contraindicated in patients with severe hepatic or renal failure, and dosage should be adjusted for those with moderate renal impairment. Notably, rivaroxaban's anticoagulant effect is not monitored via the international normalized ratio (INR), and there is no widely available method for its direct monitoring. Another option is apixaban, a direct factor Xa inhibitor, which can also serve as an alternative to rivaroxaban. According to the American College of Chest Physicians (ACCP) guidelines (10th edition, CHEST AT10), newer anticoagulants such as dabigatran, rivaroxaban, apixaban, and edoxaban are preferred over traditional vitamin K antagonists like warfarin. These alternatives eliminate the need for injections and routine monitoring of anticoagulation status, unlike warfarin, which requires frequent dose adjustments and monitoring.

Andexanet alfa, an inactivated recombinant factor Xa, has been shown to reverse the anticoagulant effects of rivaroxaban and apixaban in cases of bleeding. For cancer patients, LMWH is generally preferred over warfarin for a treatment duration of 3 to 6 months, although this decision should be based on local protocols. Regardless of the initial anticoagulation regimen, most patients will require ongoing anticoagulation for 3 to 6 months, although the optimal duration remains under debate. Management should ideally involve referral to a hematologist or vascular physician, depending on local protocols.

Graduated compression stockings for below-the-knee use have been suggested to reduce the incidence of post-phlebitic syndrome, although benefits only become apparent after two years of use, and patient tolerance is generally poor. For patients with extensive ilio-femoral thrombosis, thrombolysis should be considered, especially when hemodynamic changes suggest multiple pulmonary emboli. In cases where lower limb vital functions are at risk, thrombectomy may be necessary to reduce the risk of post-thrombotic syndrome. Systemic thrombolysis for occlusive venous thrombi is often less effective, and the risk of bleeding may outweigh its benefits. In contrast, catheter-directed thrombolytic therapy has been used with some success for large symptomatic ilio-femoral thrombosis.

Pregnant women suspected of having deep vein thrombosis (DVT) have not been extensively studied regarding diagnostic protocols, so caution is necessary. Generally, all pregnant patients should undergo compression ultrasonography, with a low threshold for initiating LMWH treatment. A dilemma arises in cases of isolated DVT below the popliteal vein or in cases of equivocal findings in the calf with negative results above the knee. Possible options include withholding anticoagulation and monitoring with serial ultrasound or starting anticoagulation therapy. The CHEST AT10 guidelines recommend anticoagulation for distal DVTs with certain risk factors, such as a positive D-dimer, extensive thrombosis, thrombosis near proximal veins, or a history of venous thromboembolism (VTE). In cases where anticoagulation is not started for infra-popliteal DVT, repeat ultrasound after 1 to 2 weeks is advised to detect any clot progression. Given the risk of clot extension and the safety of LMWH, it is often prudent to initiate anticoagulation for confirmed below-knee DVT and investigate equivocal cases further.

Thrombosis in the subclavian and axillary veins is less common than lower limb thrombosis, typically associated with an indwelling venous catheter, active cancer, or mechanical compression. This condition may also follow strenuous upper extremity exertion, such as weightlifting, though this is rare. Patients usually present with swelling of the arm, which may develop either rapidly or gradually. Symptoms often include arm heaviness and discomfort, worsened by activity and relieved by rest. Clinical findings may include increased prominence of veins, skin mottling, or non-pitting edema, along with tenderness in the axillary vein. If the internal jugular vein is enlarged, superior vena cava obstruction should be considered.

The diagnosis of upper limb DVT is most commonly made with duplex ultrasound, which is both highly sensitive and specific. Standard treatment consists of anticoagulation to prevent thrombus progression, along with rest, heat, and elevation for symptom relief. Catheter-directed thrombolysis, anticoagulation, and possibly venous angioplasty may be considered to restore vein patency. Long-term anticoagulation should only be used if recurrent thrombosis risk factors are present, such as thrombophilia.

Future Directions:

Statin therapy and other secondary prevention measures for vascular disease may influence the incidence of peripheral arterial disease, especially in developed countries. In contrast, smoking and atherogenic diets in developing countries, coupled with an aging population, may increase the incidence of cardiovascular and arterial diseases.

New anticoagulant therapies and their reversal agents are likely to impact both initial and long-term management of venous disease.

Future training may enable emergency physicians to diagnose or rule out DVT more definitively via compression ultrasound, reducing the reliance on D-dimer testing.

Controversies:

The evolving role of thrombolysis for acute arterial occlusion remains debated.

There is no clear consensus on optimal drug regimens, anticoagulation durations, and costs for treating DVT.

The management of below-knee DVT and its treatment protocols remains contentious, particularly in pregnant women, where protocols are underdeveloped.

References

1. Aboyans, V., Ricco, J. B., Bartelink, M. L., et al. (2017). ESC Guidelines on the Diagnosis and Treatment of Peripheral Arterial Diseases, in collaboration with the European Society for Vascular Surgery (ESVS). This document addresses atherosclerotic diseases of the extracranial carotid and vertebral, mesenteric, renal, and upper and lower extremity arteries. Endorsed by the European Stroke Organization (ESO) and the Task Force for the Diagnosis and Treatment of Peripheral Arterial Diseases of the

European Society of Cardiology (ESC) and the European Society for Vascular Surgery (ESVS). European Heart Journal, 39(9), 763–816.

2. Bernardi, E., Camporese, G., Büller, H. R., et al. (2008). Serial 2-point ultrasonography plus D-dimer vs. whole-leg color-coded Doppler ultrasonography for diagnosing suspected symptomatic deep vein thrombosis: A randomized controlled trial. JAMA, 300(14), 1653–1659.

3. Berridge, D. C., Kessel, D. O., & Robertson, I. (2013). Surgery versus thrombolysis for the initial management of acute limb ischemia. Cochrane Database of Systematic Reviews, 6, CD002784.

4. Duval, S., Keo, H. H., Oldenburg, N. C., et al. (2014). The impact of prolonged lower limb ischemia on amputation, mortality, and functional status: The FRIENDS registry. American Heart Journal, 168(4), 577–587.

5. Gerhard-Herman, M. D., Gornik, H. L., Barrett, C., et al. (2017). 2016 AHA/ACC guideline on the management of patients with lower extremity peripheral artery disease: Executive summary: A report of the American College of Cardiology/American Heart Association Task Force on Clinical Practice Guidelines. Circulation, 135(12), e686–e725.

6. Kearon, C., Akl, E. A., Ornelas, J., et al. (2016). Antithrombotic therapy for VTE disease: CHEST guideline and expert panel report. Chest, 149(2), 315–352.

7. Kleinjan, A., Di Nisio, M., Beyer-Westendorf, J., et al. (2014). Safety and feasibility of a diagnostic algorithm combining clinical probability, D-dimer testing, and ultrasonography for suspected upper extremity deep venous thrombosis: A prospective management study. Annals of Internal Medicine, 160(7), 451–457.

8. Linkins, L. A., Bates, S. M., Lang, E., et al. (2013). Selective D-dimer testing for diagnosis of a first suspected episode of deep venous thrombosis: A randomized trial. Annals of Internal Medicine, 158(2), 93–100.

9. NICE Guidelines CG147 (2012). Lower limb peripheral arterial disease: Full guideline. Retrieved from https://www.nice.org.uk/guidance/CG147. Accessed June 2018.

10. Wells, P. S., Owen, C., Doucette, S., et al. (2006). Does this patient have deep vein thrombosis? JAMA, 295(2).

Chapter 9
Hypertension

Essentials

1. Hypertension is diagnosed when the systolic blood pressure is ≥140 mm Hg and/or the diastolic blood pressure is ≥90 mm Hg.

2. Hypertensive crises encompass both hypertensive emergencies and hypertensive urgencies.

3. A hypertensive emergency involves end-organ damage (e.g., to the brain, cardiovascular system, or kidneys) and requires immediate intervention and hospitalization.

4. While most individuals experiencing a hypertensive emergency have a history of

chronic hypertension, it can also occur in those with previously normal blood pressure.

5. Management strategies are based on the clinical presentation, the presence of complications or coexisting conditions, and the risks associated with treatment.

6. Hypertensive encephalopathy necessitates rapid blood pressure control.

7. There is inadequate evidence to recommend aggressive blood pressure reduction in cases of acute stroke, except when thrombolytic therapy is being considered.

Introduction

Hypertension is a widespread health condition with significant implications for cardiovascular, renal, and neurological health. It is typically defined as having a systolic blood pressure of 140 mm Hg or greater and/or a diastolic blood pressure of 90 mm Hg or greater. Normal blood pressure is considered to be less than 120/80 mm Hg. While the threshold between normal and hypertensive blood pressure is useful for diagnosis and treatment decisions, it is somewhat arbitrary, and practical management often depends on these cut-off values. Hypertension is diagnosed, managed, and treated based on these criteria, which help determine when to begin screening and intervention.

Hypertensive crises, including hypertensive urgencies and emergencies, occur in a small proportion (1% to 2%) of individuals with hypertension. These are typically characterized by a diastolic blood pressure higher than 120 mm Hg. However, the importance of the absolute value of blood pressure may vary, as patients with long-standing hypertension can often tolerate higher levels compared to those with previously normal blood pressure. The critical feature of a hypertensive crisis is the presence of symptoms and/or organ damage. The term "malignant hypertension," coined in 1928, is now considered outdated due to significant advancements in treatment, which have reduced mortality rates from hypertensive emergencies from 80% to less than 10%.

Hypertensive Emergencies vs. Hypertensive Urgencies

The first step in emergency department (ED) management of hypertension is differentiating between a hypertensive emergency and an urgency. A hypertensive emergency is defined as severely elevated blood pressure (systolic >180 mm Hg and/or diastolic >120 mm Hg) with signs of organ damage, including cardiovascular, renal, or neurological complications. Immediate treatment is required to lower blood pressure in these cases, although normalization is not necessary. In contrast, hypertensive urgency refers to significantly high blood pressure without evidence of acute organ damage. Most of these patients are either non-compliant with or have discontinued antihypertensive therapy. While these cases require urgent intervention, treatment typically involves restarting or adjusting oral antihypertensive medications, with follow-up within 24 to 48 hours.

Epidemiology

Hypertension is a leading global health issue, affecting approximately 1 billion people worldwide. Studies indicate that 3% of the population develops hypertension annually, with a higher prevalence in males. Certain populations, such as Australian Indigenous peoples and African Americans, have an increased risk of developing hypertension. Approximately 30% of people with hypertension are undiagnosed, and 29% of diagnosed individuals have inadequate control over their condition.

Hypertensive Emergencies

Hypertensive emergencies can affect multiple organ systems, with the most commonly involved being the brain, heart, kidneys, and large arteries. The clinical presentation often reflects the target organ(s) involved.

Neurological Hypertensive Emergencies

Hypertensive encephalopathy is a critical neurological emergency that results from acute increases in blood pressure. The brain's autoregulatory mechanisms maintain stable cerebral blood flow within a mean arterial pressure (MAP) range of 60–120 mm Hg. When blood pressure exceeds this threshold, the body compensates by constricting blood vessels. However, once this limit is surpassed (typically MAP >180 mm Hg), the vessels dilate, leading to cerebral edema and neurological symptoms. In normotensive individuals, this may occur with blood pressure as low as 160/100 mm Hg (MAP ~120 mm Hg), whereas in chronically hypertensive patients, the autoregulatory range may shift, delaying encephalopathy. The classic triad of hypertensive encephalopathy includes severe hypertension, altered consciousness (confusion, seizures, coma), and retinopathy (retinal hemorrhages, exudates, papilledema). If not promptly treated, the condition can progress to cerebral hemorrhage, edema, or death. High-risk groups include individuals with untreated hypertension, kidney disease, or certain medications like erythropoietin.

Ischemic stroke patients often present with elevated blood pressure, observed in up to 80% of cases. While high blood pressure in the acute phase generally resolves within 90 minutes, its effect on long-term outcomes is still debated. Hemorrhagic stroke, particularly intracerebral and subarachnoid, is also associated with elevated blood pressure, which can exacerbate hematoma expansion and worsen prognosis, especially when systolic blood pressure exceeds 200 mm Hg.

Cardiovascular Hypertensive Emergencies

Common cardiovascular emergencies related to hypertension include acute pulmonary edema, acute coronary syndrome, and aortic dissection.

Acute pulmonary edema occurs when elevated blood pressure leads to left ventricular dysfunction, increasing myocardial oxygen demand. This condition is a frequent manifestation of hypertensive emergencies.

Acute coronary syndrome arises when elevated systemic vascular resistance increases myocardial wall tension and oxygen demand, leading to ischemia, particularly in patients with pre-existing coronary artery disease.

Acute aortic dissection is a rare but life-threatening condition, often presenting with chest pain and hypertension. It is characterized by a tear in the aortic wall and can lead to rapid deterioration.

Renal Hypertensive Emergencies

Severe hypertension can directly damage the kidneys, resulting in hypertensive nephrosclerosis, or it may exacerbate underlying kidney disease. Chronic renal failure, particularly in patients requiring dialysis or those with a history of kidney transplants, can lead to a cycle of escalating blood pressure and worsening renal function.

Hypertensive Emergencies in Pregnancy

Pre-eclampsia is a significant hypertensive disorder in pregnancy, characterized by hypertension (≥140/90 mm Hg) and evidence of end-organ damage after 20 weeks of gestation. This condition poses significant risks to both maternal and fetal health.

Clinical Evaluation of Hypertensive Crisis

A thorough clinical assessment is essential in identifying end-organ dysfunction and establishing the underlying cause of hypertension. Key areas of evaluation include:

Blood pressure measurement (preferably in both arms)

Cardiovascular examination (peripheral pulses, signs of cardiac failure, renal bruits)

Neurological examination and fundoscopy (retinal hemorrhages, papilledema)

Investigations

Investigation should be guided by the clinical presentation. Key tests include:

Electrocardiography (ECG), especially if chest pain is present, to assess for left ventricular hypertrophy or ischemia.

Urinalysis to check for hematuria and proteinuria.

Blood tests to assess renal function, electrolytes, and detect secondary causes of hypertension.

Imaging, such as chest x-rays or cerebral CT scans, may be necessary to rule out complications like pulmonary edema or hemorrhagic stroke.

Treatment

The main goal in managing hypertensive emergencies is to prevent further organ damage. Blood pressure should be reduced cautiously to avoid hypoperfusion of critical organs. In general, the mean arterial pressure (MAP) should be lowered by no more than 25% in the first hour, aiming for a target of <180/120 mm Hg. Over the next 23 hours, further reduction to <160/110 mm Hg is ideal, except in cases like aortic dissection, severe pre-eclampsia, or pheochromocytoma crisis, where rapid blood pressure reduction is necessary. Parenteral antihypertensive agents are recommended, with the patient closely monitored in a resuscitation setting, ideally with intra-arterial blood pressure monitoring.

While there is limited high-quality evidence to guide treatment, management guidelines are largely consensus-based, and therapy must be tailored to the specific clinical scenario.

Hypertensive Urgency: Evaluation and Treatment

Management of markedly elevated blood pressure (BP) in the emergency department (ED) without signs of end-organ damage remains unclear. The initial assessment follows similar steps as hypertensive emergencies, focusing on ruling out end-organ dysfunction through a thorough history and physical examination. There is debate about whether routine investigations should be conducted due to the absence of large randomized clinical trials. Available evidence suggests that screening for serum creatinine levels in the ED can identify a small group of patients with renal dysfunction, but it is uncertain how this compares to patients with normal or near-normal BP. No additional diagnostic tests seem to provide useful information.

The decision to treat asymptomatic patients in the ED is also challenging due to the lack of high-quality evidence. However, several consensus guidelines suggest gradual BP reduction (within hours to days) to a target of <160/100 mm Hg or a reduction of 25-30% from baseline. This approach aims to avoid the risks of stroke or myocardial infarction if the BP is lowered too much, especially in individuals with pre-existing hypertension. Treatment strategies often begin with a "wait-and-treat" approach, where the patient rests for 30 minutes or longer in a quiet room, potentially reducing BP by more than 20/10 mm Hg in about one-third of cases. If BP remains elevated, oral antihypertensive treatment is appropriate. Given that most hypertensive patients are noncompliant with medications, restarting their regular medications is recommended if this issue is identified.

Angiotensin-converting enzyme inhibitors (ACEIs) are often first-line treatments in these patients.

Disposition of patients depends on comorbidities, response to treatment, and the availability of follow-up care within 24-48 hours.

Prognosis and Disposition

The prognosis for hypertensive urgency depends on how effectively treatment prevents further end-organ damage. Patients with hypertensive emergencies require admission to a high-dependency area with invasive blood pressure monitoring. In contrast, patients with hypertensive urgency who are suitable for discharge must have follow-up within 48 hours. Those with high-risk features or significant comorbidities should be observed in the hospital.

Future Developments

Emerging research may improve our understanding of the triggers for hypertensive emergencies. Specifically, evidence suggesting that intensive lifelong management with a target BP of 120/80 mm Hg could reduce cardiovascular disease risk significantly. Furthermore, increasing evidence supports the use of home automated BP monitoring in clinical practice, which may become a more integral part of patient care.

Controversies

The management of elevated blood pressure in the acute phase of a stroke remains controversial. There is no consensus on when to treat or the timing of intervention, and each case should be evaluated individually.

There is also a lack of robust evidence regarding the overall benefit of antihypertensive drugs and the choice of first-line therapy in hypertensive emergencies, primarily due to small trial sizes, lack of long-term follow-up, and methodological challenges.

References

1. Cherney D, Straus S. Management of patients with hypertensive urgencies and emergencies—a systematic review of the literature. J Gen Intern Med. 2002;17(12):937-945.

2. Feldstein C. Management of hypertensive crises. Am J Ther. 2007;14:138-139.

3. Johnson W, Nguyen ML, Patel R. Hypertension crisis in the emergency department. Cardiol Clin. 2012;30:533.

4. Lowe SA, Bowyer L, Lust K, et al. SOMANZ guidelines for the management of hypertensive disorders of pregnancy 2014. Aust N Z J Obstet Gynaecol. 2015;55(5):e1-e29.

5. Papadopoulos DP, Sanidas EA, Viniou NA, et al. Cardiovascular hypertensive emergencies. Curr Hypertens Rep. 2015;17(2):5.

6. Shayne PH, Pitts SR. Severely increased blood pressure in the emergency department. Ann Emerg Med. 2003;41(4):513-529.

7. Stroke Foundation. Clinical Guidelines for Stroke Management 2017. Melbourne; 2017.

8. Vaughan CJ, Delanty N. Hypertensive emergencies. Lancet. 2000;356(9227):4411-4417.

9. Whelton PK, Carey RM, Aronow WS, et al. 2017 ACC/AHA Guideline for the prevention, detection, evaluation, and management of high blood pressure in adults. J Am Coll Cardiol. 2018;71(19):e127-e248.

10. Wolf SJ, Lo B, Shih RD, et al. American College of Emergency Physicians Clinical Policies Committee. Clinical policy: critical

issues in the evaluation and management of adult patients in the emergency department with asymptomatic elevated blood pressure. Ann Emerg Med. 2013;62(1):59-68.

Chapter 10
Aortic dissection

Essentials

1. Mortality and Early Management: Without treatment, aortic dissection has a mortality rate of approximately 1% per hour during the first 48 hours, with a 90% mortality rate within three months. However, early detection and prompt treatment can reduce mortality to 20%-40%.

2. Diagnosis: Aortic dissection is a rare condition that requires a high level of suspicion and targeted diagnostic investigation for confirmation.

3. Diagnostic Errors: Both false-negative and false-positive diagnoses of aortic dissection can lead to higher morbidity and mortality rates.

4. Imaging: In unstable patients, transesophageal echocardiography (TEE) is the preferred

imaging method. For stable patients, computed tomography aortography (CTA) is the imaging modality of choice when aortic dissection is suspected.

5. Initial Therapy: Treatment to lower blood pressure and reduce the force of ventricular contraction should begin as soon as aortic dissection is suspected.

6. Management: Proximal dissections typically require immediate surgery, while uncomplicated distal dissections are generally managed with medical treatment. Complicated distal dissections are often treated with endoluminal stenting or surgery.

Introduction

Aortic dissection (AD) is a rare but potentially fatal condition. Its diverse clinical presentation requires a high level of suspicion for early diagnosis. Rapid and targeted investigations are crucial for confirming the diagnosis, as the mortality rate for untreated AD can be as high as 1% per hour during the first 48 hours. AD is a part of acute aortic syndrome, which includes several severe aortic conditions such as intramural hematoma, penetrating aortic ulcer, and traumatic aortic transection. All these conditions share a common pathophysiological endpoint: the separation of the aortic intima from the outer aortic layers, leading to devastating outcomes. The signs, symptoms, and management strategies for these conditions exhibit considerable overlap.

Epidemiology, Pathophysiology, and Classification

The incidence of aortic dissection is approximately 3 cases per 100,000 individuals annually. Up to half of the cases are only detected at autopsy. Despite its low overall incidence, aortic dissection is the most frequent catastrophic aortic event, occurring two to three times more often than abdominal aortic rupture. The condition predominantly affects males, particularly those aged between 50 and 70. Proximal dissections (involving the aortic arch) typically occur about 10 years earlier than distal dissections. Risk factors for AD include hypertension, which is the most significant, and a history of Marfan syndrome, which accounts for approximately 5% of cases.

AD typically results from two key factors: arterial hypertension and the degeneration of the aortic media. Dissection occurs when blood is forced into a low-resistance tissue plane in the aortic wall, caused by a weakened media. Two mechanisms have been proposed for initiating the dissection. The traditional theory suggests an intimal tear, typically occurring near areas of high hydrodynamic stress, such as above the aortic valve or at the ligamentum . This tear allows high-pressure blood to infiltrate the aortic media, creating a false lumen that may extend either proximally or distally. An alternative theory posits that ruptured vasa within the media lead to the formation of an intramural hematoma, which can expand and eventually tear the intima. Interestingly, autopsy studies show that 12% of dissections lack an identifiable intimal tear, indicating it may not always be a prerequisite for the condition.

The progression of dissection can involve the occlusion of branch vessels, resulting in ischemia and organ dysfunction. Proximal dissections may cause aortic valve insufficiency, and further extension can lead to pericardial tamponade. The false lumen created by the dissection may obstruct the true lumen or rupture outward, leading to exsanguination. External rupture is most commonly observed in the left pleural cavity or mediastinum. The rate of dissection propagation is influenced by the patient's blood pressure and the gradient of the arterial pressure wave, making blood pressure reduction a key therapeutic target.

Classification

The Stanford and De Bakey classification systems are commonly used to categorize aortic dissections based on their anatomical features. The Stanford system divides dissections into two types: Type A, which involves the ascending aorta (with or without the descending aorta), and Type B, which is limited to the descending aorta. This system is widely used due to its simplicity. The De Bakey system is more detailed, with Type I involving both the ascending and descending aorta, Type II affecting only the ascending aorta, and Type III involving only the descending aorta (subdivided into Type IIIa and Type IIIb based on thoracic and abdominal involvement). Additionally, aortic dissection is classified as acute if symptoms last less than 14 days, or chronic if they persist longer than 14 days.

Clinical Features

Pain is the hallmark symptom of aortic dissection, affecting 74% to 95% of patients. The pain is often described as severe, tearing, or ripping, and is usually maximal at onset. It may migrate depending on the dissection's progression. Pain from ascending aortic involvement is typically felt in the anterior chest, while descending aorta involvement causes interscapular pain that can extend to the back or abdomen as the dissection progresses distally.

Other symptoms arise from complications such as branch vessel occlusion. Up to 20% of patients may present with coma, confusion, or stroke due to carotid artery involvement or inadequate perfusion from shock. Neurological symptoms may fluctuate, and 2% to 8% of patients experience paraplegia or paraesthesia due to spinal artery separation. Syncope, especially in Type A dissections, can suggest rupture into the pericardium.

Other less common symptoms result from local compression due to contained rupture, such as superior vena cava syndrome, hoarseness, dyspnea, dysphagia, upper airway obstruction, or Horner syndrome. A thorough risk factor assessment is essential for diagnosis.

Examination

There is no single examination finding that can confirm aortic dissection, and patients typically appear acutely distressed, with pain resistant to analgesics. Tachycardia is common, reflecting pain, anxiety, and shock. Hypertension occurs in 50% to 78% of patients, especially those with Type B dissection, either due to pre-existing hypertension or as an acute response to pain. Hypotension is a critical sign, indicating potential aortic rupture or pericardial tamponade.

Signs of side branch occlusion may include neurological deficits, limb ischemia, or pulse differences between the upper limbs. Proximal dissection may lead to acute aortic incompetence, possibly causing acute left ventricular failure. A diastolic murmur indicative of aortic incompetence is common in proximal dissections, and pericardial tamponade may present with the Beck triad: hypotension, muffled heart sounds, and elevated jugular venous pressure. Pulsus or a pericardial friction rub may also be detected. Renal artery involvement may result in oliguria or anuria.

Clinical Investigations

Initial investigations should focus on excluding other diagnoses or increasing suspicion of aortic dissection. Routine blood tests are not diagnostic but can establish baseline values such as renal function and hemoglobin levels. An electrocardiogram (ECG) is essential to rule out acute myocardial infarction, as up to 40% of aortic dissection patients show signs suggestive of ischemia. ECG abnormalities may also indicate coronary artery involvement, though this is relatively rare.

Chest X-ray (CXR) may show abnormalities in 72% to 90% of cases, but its sensitivity and specificity are low. A normal CXR should not rule out dissection. Specific imaging tests, including computed tomography (CT), echocardiography, aortography, and magnetic resonance imaging (MRI), are required to confirm the diagnosis, determine the dissection's location, and assess complications. These tests should be performed promptly, with the choice of modality depending on patient stability, test availability, and institutional protocols.

Aortic Dissection Management

MRI and its Limitations in Acute Management

Magnetic resonance imaging (MRI) provides detailed insights into aortic dissection; however, it is not suitable for patients who are unstable or at risk of becoming unstable. This limitation is due to the need for immediate stabilization and resuscitation in such cases. MRI is better suited for long-term monitoring or ongoing evaluation of conditions such as aortic dissection rather than for initial diagnostic purposes in acute settings.

Biomarkers for Early Detection

The use of biomarkers, particularly D-dimer, for early identification of aortic dissection is gaining attention. A 2010 meta-analysis, which evaluated D-dimer's diagnostic role, concluded that it should not be considered a standalone "rule-out" test for aortic dissection. While it holds potential, further prospective trials are required to fully understand its role in the diagnostic process. Currently, no single biomarker has been validated for diagnosing acute aortic dissection, and the potential of combination biomarker panels remains uninvestigated.

Differential Diagnosis of Aortic Dissection

Diagnosing aortic dissection is complex due to its wide-ranging symptoms and signs, making the differential diagnosis extensive. With the introduction of thrombolysis for acute embolic stroke, it is essential to rule out aortic dissection as a potential stroke mimic before administering thrombolytic agents. This underscores the importance of advanced imaging protocols, such as CT perfusion, which extends from the aortic arch to aid in identifying aortic dissection in patients presenting with suspected stroke.

Initial Treatment Strategy

The management of aortic dissection begins with immediate resuscitation, stabilization, and interventions to prevent the progression of the dissection. Timely action is critical: diagnosis and intervention should occur simultaneously, particularly in unstable patients. Early diagnosis, effective blood pressure and heart rate control, and prompt surgical intervention are key to improving survival outcomes. As aortic dissection often presents with severe pain, adequate pain relief through titrated IV narcotics should be prioritized, as pain management also contributes to lowering blood pressure and heart rate.

Pharmacological Control of Pulsatile Load

To minimize ongoing dissection, pharmacological treatment focuses on reducing the pulsatile load exerted by the left ventricle onto the false lumen. This load is influenced by systolic blood pressure and the velocity of ventricular ejection. The goal is to reduce blood pressure without increasing heart rate or contractility. Beta-blockers, such as esmolol (a short-acting agent), are ideal for their negative inotropic and chronotropic effects. Esmolol is typically administered via a loading infusion followed by a maintenance infusion. If esmolol is unavailable, metoprolol is a suitable alternative. Blood pressure targets generally aim for a systolic range of 100–120 mm Hg and a heart rate between 60 and 80 beats per minute. Intra-arterial monitoring is crucial for precise blood pressure management.

For further blood pressure reduction, vasodilators like sodium nitroprusside or glyceryl trinitrate (GTN) may be utilized. Sodium nitroprusside works by systemic vasodilation and has a rapid onset and short duration of action. However, the risk of cyanide toxicity limits its use to 24 hours. GTN, more commonly used, reduces both preload and afterload but may induce reflex tachycardia, which requires prior β-blockade.

Management of Type A Aortic Dissection

Open surgical repair is the preferred treatment for acute type A aortic dissection, especially for preventing rupture and restoring blood flow to affected regions. The surgery typically involves excising the affected aortic segment and replacing it with a prosthetic graft. Despite its potential benefits, surgical mortality for type A dissection ranges from 5% to 21%. Without surgery, the mortality rate for acute type A dissection can reach up to 90% within 3 months. Post-surgical survival at 5 years ranges from 56% to 87%.

Management of Type B Aortic Dissection

Type B aortic dissections are classified as either complicated (30%) or uncomplicated (70%). Uncomplicated cases can often be managed medically with tight blood pressure and heart rate control, leading to an 80% survival rate after 1 year. The role of endoluminal stenting for uncomplicated cases has not been shown to improve long-term survival outcomes when compared to medical management alone.

Complicated type B dissections, which include risks such as rupture or end-organ ischemia, were historically managed by open surgery, with high mortality rates (21% to 33.9%). The advent of endovascular stent grafts has significantly reduced both mortality and morbidity, improving outcomes for patients with complicated type B dissections. However, a notable portion of these patients may require additional procedures. In-hospital mortality has decreased to 10%, and major morbidity, including renal failure and stroke, has halved compared to open surgical repair.

All patients with aortic dissection, whether treated medically or surgically, are typically placed on lifelong β-blockade. Serial MRI imaging is essential for long-term monitoring of the aorta.

Prognosis

Survival rates for aortic dissection have improved significantly over the past few decades due to advances in both medical and surgical interventions. One-year survival rates are reported at 52% to 69% for type A dissection and around 70% for type B dissection. The most common cause of death in aortic dissection is rupture, particularly into the pericardial sac, while multi-organ failure also contributes to mortality following treatment.

Disposition and Follow-Up Care

Patients who do not require emergency surgery should be admitted to intensive care for monitoring and aggressive management to prevent further dissection progression. In cases where patients are in peripheral or regional centers, transfer to a specialized cardiothoracic unit is necessary once their condition has been stabilized.

Controversies in Aortic Dissection Management

The role of intravascular ultrasound in diagnosis, while having high sensitivity and specificity, has not been proven practical in the emergency department setting.

The utility of chest X-rays (CXR) as a screening tool for aortic dissection remains limited.

The use of D-dimers as a rule-out test in low-risk patients is still under debate.

Preventive strategies for Marfan syndrome, such as routine β-blockade and elective grafting of the aortic valve and ascending aorta, are being discussed for patients at high risk.

References

1. Ahmad F, Cheshire N, Hamady M. Acute aortic syndrome: pathology and therapeutic strategies. Postgrad Med J. 2006;82:305–312.

2. Hagan PG, Nienaber CA, Isselbacher EM, et al. The International Registry of

Dissection (IRAD): new insights into an old disease. JAMA. 2000;283(7):897–903.

3. Nienaber CA, Rousseau H, Eggebrecht H, et al. Randomised comparison of strategies for type B aortic dissection: the INvestigation of STEnt Grafts in Aortic Dissection (INSTEAD) trial. Circulation. 2009;120:2519–2528.

4. Trimarchi S, Nienaber CA, Rampoldi V, et al. Role and results of surgery in acute type B aortic dissection: insights from the International Registry of Acute Aortic Dissection (IRAD). Circulation. 2006;114:1357–1364.

Glossary

Acute Coronary Syndrome (ACS)
An umbrella term for conditions resulting from a sudden reduction in blood flow to the heart, including unstable angina, NSTEMI, and STEMI. It requires immediate medical intervention.

Acute Myocardial Infarction (AMI)
A medical condition where there is a sudden blockage of a coronary artery, leading to damage or death of heart muscle tissue due to the lack of blood flow and oxygen.

Advanced Cardiovascular Life Support (ACLS)
A set of clinical interventions used to manage cardiac arrest, stroke, and other cardiovascular emergencies, focusing on life-threatening arrhythmias, airway management, and medication administration.

Ablation Therapy

A medical procedure used to treat abnormal heart rhythms (arrhythmias) by destroying or scarring the tissue responsible for the irregular electrical signals.

Aortic Dissection
A serious condition in which a tear occurs in the inner layer of the aorta, leading to a separation of the layers of the arterial wall, causing pain and potentially fatal complications.

Aortic Occlusion and Resuscitation Therapy for Acute (AORTA)
A procedure used in cases of severe hemorrhagic shock to provide controlled occlusion of the aorta, improving perfusion to vital organs.

Angina Pectoris
Chest pain caused by reduced blood flow to the heart muscle, often due to coronary artery disease.

Angiotensin-Converting Enzyme (ACE) Inhibitors

A class of drugs that relax blood vessels and lower blood pressure by inhibiting the enzyme that produces angiotensin II, a substance that narrows blood vessels.

Angiotensin II Receptor Blockers (ARBs)
Medications that block the effects of angiotensin II, helping to lower blood pressure and reduce strain on the heart.

Anticoagulants
Drugs that prevent blood clot formation by inhibiting the coagulation cascade, commonly used in the treatment of acute coronary syndrome, atrial fibrillation, and venous thromboembolism.

Antiplatelet Therapy
Medications, such as aspirin or clopidogrel, that prevent platelets from aggregating and forming clots, are often used in the treatment of acute coronary syndromes and to prevent stroke.

Arterial Blood Gas (ABG)

A test that measures the levels of oxygen, carbon dioxide, and pH in the blood, used to assess respiratory function and metabolic state in critically ill patients.

Baroreceptor Reflex
A physiological mechanism in which the body adjusts blood pressure by changing heart rate and vessel tone in response to detected changes in blood pressure.

Beta-Blockers
A class of medications that reduce heart rate and blood pressure by blocking the effects of adrenaline on the heart, commonly used in the management of hypertension, heart failure, and arrhythmias.

Cardiogenic Shock
A life-threatening condition in which the heart is unable to pump enough blood to meet the body's needs, often resulting from a severe heart attack or other heart failure conditions.

Cardiopulmonary Bypass (CPB)
A technique used during heart surgery where a machine temporarily takes over the function of the heart and lungs to circulate and oxygenate blood while the heart is being repaired.

Cardiopulmonary Resuscitation (CPR)
A life-saving technique performed on individuals who are in cardiac arrest, involving chest compressions and, if necessary, artificial ventilation.

Cardiovascular Emergency
A life-threatening condition involving the heart and/or blood vessels, requiring immediate medical intervention, such as myocardial infarction, stroke, and severe arrhythmias.

Chronic Obstructive Pulmonary Disease (COPD)
A progressive lung disease that can worsen the symptoms of cardiovascular emergencies, particularly in patients with heart failure, leading to further complications.

Coronary Artery Bypass Grafting (CABG)
A surgical procedure used to treat coronary artery disease by diverting blood flow around a blocked or narrowed artery in the heart.

Culprit Lesion
The specific blocked or narrowed artery responsible for causing an acute myocardial infarction or other acute coronary syndrome.

Defibrillation
The use of an electric shock to restore a normal heart rhythm in patients experiencing certain arrhythmias, such as ventricular fibrillation or pulseless ventricular tachycardia.

Defibrillator
A device used to deliver a controlled electric shock to the heart to restore a normal rhythm in cases of life-threatening arrhythmias such as ventricular fibrillation.

Dopamine

A medication used to treat shock and severe hypotension, acting as a vasopressor to increase heart rate and blood pressure. It also has inotropic effects that help improve cardiac output.

Ductus Arteriosus
A fetal blood vessel that connects the pulmonary artery to the aorta. Normally closes after birth, but in certain conditions, it may remain open, leading to circulatory issues in neonates.

Electrocardiogram (ECG/EKG)
A diagnostic tool that records the electrical activity of the heart, often used to identify arrhythmias, myocardial infarctions, and other cardiovascular conditions.

Echocardiogram
An imaging technique that uses ultrasound waves to create images of the heart, allowing healthcare providers to assess heart function, valve issues, and other cardiac conditions.

Endothelial Dysfunction
A condition where the endothelial cells that line the blood vessels do not function normally, often contributing to the development of atherosclerosis and other cardiovascular diseases.

Extracorporeal Membrane Oxygenation (ECMO)
A life-support machine used in patients with severe cardiac or respiratory failure, providing long-term oxygenation and support to the heart and lungs when they are unable to function.

Fibrinolytics
Medications that break down fibrin in blood clots, used in the treatment of myocardial infarction and stroke to restore blood flow in blocked arteries.

Heart Failure (HF)
A condition in which the heart is unable to pump blood efficiently, leading to insufficient oxygen and nutrient delivery to tissues and organs.

Heart Rate Variability (HRV)
The variation in time between consecutive heartbeats, which can be an indicator of autonomic nervous system function and cardiovascular health.

Hemodynamic Monitoring
The measurement and assessment of the cardiovascular system's function, including blood pressure, heart rate, and cardiac output, often using invasive methods.

Hemorrhagic Shock
A type of shock resulting from significant blood loss, leading to inadequate perfusion of vital organs. It is often managed with blood transfusions and volume resuscitation.

Hyperkalemia
An elevated level of potassium in the blood, which can cause arrhythmias and is commonly seen in patients with kidney failure or those on

certain medications like ACE inhibitors or potassium-sparing diuretics.

Hypertensive Crisis
A severe increase in blood pressure that can lead to organ damage, including the brain, kidneys, and heart. It requires immediate intervention to lower blood pressure.

Hypertrophic Cardiomyopathy (HCM)
A genetic condition where the heart muscle becomes abnormally thick, leading to a risk of arrhythmias, sudden cardiac arrest, and heart failure.

Intra-Aortic Balloon Pump (IABP)
A device used to support the heart in cases of cardiogenic shock by inflating and deflating a balloon in the aorta to increase blood flow to the coronary arteries.

Ischemic Stroke

A type of stroke caused by a blockage in one of the arteries supplying blood to the brain, leading to tissue damage and neurological deficits.

Intravenous (IV) Therapy
The administration of fluids, medications, or nutrients directly into a vein to treat dehydration, infections, or other acute conditions.

Left Ventricular (LV) Dysfunction
A condition in which the left ventricle of the heart does not contract properly, often due to myocardial infarction or heart failure, resulting in decreased cardiac output.

Left Ventricular Assist Device (LVAD)
A mechanical pump used to support heart function in patients with severe heart failure, helping the heart pump blood to the rest of the body.

Myocardial Infarction (MI)

Commonly known as a heart attack, it occurs when blood flow to a part of the heart muscle is blocked, causing tissue damage.

Natriuretic Peptides
Hormones released by the heart in response to excessive stretching of heart muscle cells, often elevated in heart failure and used as biomarkers for diagnosis and monitoring.

Nitroglycerin
A medication that dilates blood vessels, reducing the workload of the heart and improving blood flow. It is commonly used in the treatment of angina and acute myocardial infarction.

Percutaneous Coronary Intervention (PCI)
A non-surgical procedure used to treat coronary artery disease by inserting a catheter into the artery to open blockages, often with the placement of a stent to keep the artery open.

Pharmacologic Resuscitation

The use of medications to support cardiovascular function during an emergency, including drugs to manage blood pressure, heart rate, and arrhythmias.

Preload

The initial stretching of the heart muscle fibers before contraction, related to the volume of blood entering the heart during diastole.

Pulmonary Edema

A condition in which excess fluid accumulates in the lungs, often caused by heart failure, leading to impaired gas exchange and difficulty breathing.

Pulmonary Embolism (PE)

A blockage of one of the pulmonary arteries in the lungs, typically caused by a blood clot that has traveled from the legs (deep vein thrombosis) or other parts of the body (venous thromboembolism).

Reperfusion Therapy

Treatment aimed at restoring blood flow to the heart muscle, such as thrombolysis (clot-busting drugs) or percutaneous coronary interventions

www.ingramcontent.com/pod-product-compliance
Lightning Source LLC
Chambersburg PA
CBHW071446220526
45472CB00003B/687